COLLINS POCKET REFERENCE

PRESCRIPTION DRUGS

Robert M. Youngson

HarperCollins*Publishers*

HarperCollins Publishers
P.O. Box, Glasgow G4 0NB

First published 1994

Reprint 10 9 8 7 6 5 4 3 2 1 0

© Robert M. Youngson 1994

ISBN 0 00 470535 1

Produced by Maury-Eurolivres S.A.
45300 Manchecourt - France

CONTENTS

Acknowledgements

A book of this kind can hardly be written without some errors creeping into the manuscript. Happily, however, I have had the benefit of a great deal of careful and critical checking by two distinguished medical experts, Dr S G Owen and Dr R Jalan. For their corrections, comments, amendments and helpful suggestions, I am most grateful. I wish, also, to express my grateful thanks to Gail Strachan, my meticulous and tactful editor at HarperCollins.

1. THE STORY OF DRUGS

This book is intended to be a handy reference rather than the kind of book you would want to read through like a novel. Even so, it contains a great deal of information that you are likely to find interesting for its own sake. You will also find that a basic understanding of drugs will clarify much that you have probably found obscure or confusing about medical matters generally. In addition, it will make it much easier for you to discuss your medical problems intelligently with your doctor. He or she will at once recognize that you know something about the subject, and may even spend a little more time with you than usual.

The history of drugs is fascinating, but it is also an excellent way to begin your study of drugs. The more you learn about drugs and about how they work, the more benefit you will get from this book.

The beginnings

The drug business started by accident. Early peoples, hungry or just curious, were often surprised when they sampled certain plants. Some of these caused alarming symptoms, even death. The berries of the deadly nightshade, *Atropa belladonna*, caused the unwary to develop blurred vision, dry mouth, red skin, convulsions and occasionally a fatal coma. *Cascara sagrada* beans caused alarming purgation. Chewing the leaves of the coca plant *Erythroxylum coca* caused numbing of the mouth, but relieved hunger and tiredness and made people feel happy. Eating the bark of the cinchona tree, *Cinchona succirubra*, caused excitement, confusion, singing in the ears and deafness, and caused pregnant women to lose their babies. Certain mushrooms produced extraordinary mental effects. Eating grain contaminated with rust fungus, *Claviceps purpurea*, caused gangrene and loss of legs or arms. From the earliest times, alcohol from naturally fermented grapes must have been used to relieve the frightfulness of primitive life.

These accidental discoveries were quickly exploited by the tribal healers and witch doctors and this led to a primitive tradition of drug treatment. The ancient Egyptians knew all about opium and how useful it was to relieve severe pain. They also knew that purgation with castor oil was a great help in getting rid of worms. Roman and Greek physicians used crude extracts of deadly nightshade plant, knowing that these were highly effective in relieving severe bowel colic. These extracts contained the drugs atropine (Belladonna), hyoscyamus, and stramonium, all remarkably effective in relieving muscle spasm and all still in use today. Arab physicians in the 12th century dosed their goitre patients with burnt sponges – thereby supplying essential iodine. This must often have been effective. By the 16th century doctors were giving autumn crocus (containing the alkaloid colchicine) to their gouty patients. Today's doctors still rely heavily on crocus for gout.

Magical remedies, however, persisted for a long time. As late as 1700, apothecaries were still dispensing the widely-approved cure-all, the Elixir Universale. This was a mixture of powdered lion's heart, dried human brains, gold, witch hazel, earthworms, and Egyptian onions. As today, the most powerful and effective of these early remedies were also the most dangerous. Since there was then no accurate way of knowing the strength of the active ingredient, many people must have found the treatment worse than the disease. There is no telling how many patients were poisoned or killed off by early drug treatment.

The herbals

It has never been a good idea to rely on casual word of mouth and hearsay for recommendations about drugs – especially powerful drugs. So, at an early stage, interested people started to write down what they knew about the subject. Books containing this information were called medical herbals, and a great deal of valuable knowledge about drugs, together with a considerable amount of nonsense, was preserved in this way. Some of the facts recorded in herbals were remarkable. The foxglove, *Digitalis purpurea* was widely recommended and used for the dropsy (fluid accumulation or oedema) long before Dr William Withering published his account in 1785 of the action of the dried seeds on the heart. Today every doctor knows that the oedema of heart failure can be helped by the action of digitalis in improving the efficiency of the heart. The most celebrated of the herbalists, Nicholas Culpeper (1616-1654), was also one of the most cautious. Writing of the foxglove, he warns 'The operation of this herb is often violent even in small doses: it is best not to meddle with it, lest the cure should end in the churchyard.'

The most popular natural remedies, especially those with no immediate tendency to kill off the patient, were enthusiastically taken up by doctors and others and were soon being recommended for all sorts of improbable purposes. Laudanum (tincture of opium), a solution of opium in alcohol, while obviously a powerful pain-killer and tranquillizer, was, until 100 years ago, widely recommended and used for the treatment of just about everything from toothache to tuberculosis. Millions became addicted on the orders of their doctors.

Although vitamins were not recognized until the 20th century, scurvy in sailors was effectively treated with citrus fruit as early as 1753 by James Lind (1716-1794). After Lind had presented his proof to the Admiralty, it took Their Lordships 50 years to decide to issue orders that all British sailors should have regular doses of lime juice. Meantime hundreds died of scurvy.

Morphine and pain control

The pain-relieving and mood-elevating effects of opium have been known for many thousands of years. Homer (8th c. BC) referred to a drug 'nepenthe' which was almost certainly opium. Opium is derived from the juice oozing out of cuts made in the wall of the unripe seed pod of the poppy *Papaver somniferum* soon after the petals fall. The juice dries to form a dark gummy solid which is crude opium. The word derives from a Greek root meaning 'sap' or 'juice'. The method of obtaining the drug was first recorded by Dioscorides (born around AD 50) in the first century AD and all the major medical writers throughout history have proclaimed its virtues.

Opium contains more than twenty natural drugs, including codeine, papaverine and morphine, and it is morphine which is responsible for its most important effects. It abolishes pain, hunger and thirst, eases anxiety and depression and induces sleep.

Morphine was first isolated by the German chemist Frederich Serturner (1783-1841) in 1805.

Morphine is chemically almost identical to the endorphins. These are pain-killing substances that occur naturally in the human body. Both morphine and the endorphins work by fitting into certain chemical receptor sites on nerve cells in the brain and spinal cord. This fact makes morphine a rather special drug and accounts for its uniquely effective properties in relieving pain and distress. Although many similar synthetic drugs have been developed, most doctors are agreed that there is no real substitute for morphine. Doctors now generally accept that, for patients suffering severe pain, proper dosage of morphine, even when given over long periods, need not lead to addiction. Abuse of morphine is, of course, widespread, especially in the form of heroin, which is easily made from it (see Chapter 5).

The story of quinine

Throughout recorded history, malaria has killed millions of people and caused immeasurable life-long debility. Even today it claims millions of lives every year. But as early as the 16th century the natives of Peru were aware that a bitter solution obtained from the bark of a certain tree was an effective treatment for the disease. The knowledge of this remedy was brought to Europe in 1640 by the Countess of Chincon, the wife of the Viceroy of Peru, who had been cured of an intermittent fever with the drug in the Palace of Lima. Large quantities of the bark were sent to Rome later in the century by Jesuit fathers and it came to be known as 'Jesuits' bark'. In 1742 Linnaeus (1707-1778) named the plant genus *Cinchona* in honour of the Countess.

The English physician Thomas Sydenham (1624-1698) became interested in cinchona bark and studied its properties. At first, the drug was used indiscriminately for any acute feverish illness and there were many failures. But, as the clinical features of malaria became clearer and it was more easily distinguished from other diseases, doctors realized that a major advance in treatment had been discovered. Later the active ingredient, the alkaloid quinine, was isolated and more accurate dosage became possible. Until well into the 20th century, quinine was the only available remedy or preventive for malaria.

Ergot

Farmers have long been familiar with the various fungus 'smuts' and 'rusts' that grow on grain crops. One of the most notorious of these is *Claviceps purpurea*, the fungus that grows on the fruiting spike of rye. *Claviceps* gets into the rye in the form of spores that have been lying dormant in the ground. As the plant grows the fungus destroys the rye ovary and replaces the normal grain with a black growth called an ergot. The dangers of eating rye contaminated with ergot have been known since at least 600 BC. An Assyrian tablet of the time warns against it. From the Middle Ages onwards there are numerous records of the disease known as St Anthony's Fire – a disorder featuring confusion, drowsiness, headache, seizures, severe burning pain or tingling in the extremities followed by gangrene, abortion in pregnant women and death.

All these effects are due to a tight closure of arteries from spasm of the muscles in their walls. This is caused by one of the active principles of ergot. Closure of arteries means that parts of the body are deprived of blood. Arms and legs become cold and black as the tissues die, then either shrivel or drop off. In spite of these known dangers, midwives had, for hundreds of years, been using small doses of ergot to bring on labour and strengthen contractions of the womb.

Ergot contains many powerful drugs, but it was not until the early 20th century that the first medically useful of these substances was isolated. Ergot drugs include ergotoxine (isolated in 1906), ergotamine, ergotaminine, and ergometrine. The latter drug is still used in childbirth and in the treatment of migraine. Ergometrine is now mainly restricted to use in the control of bleeding from the womb after the delivery of the baby and placenta (post-partum haemorrhage) and it has to be used with care in migraine. Because of its general effect in constricting arteries, it can be very dangerous in people with angina or narrowing of the limb arteries (peripheral vascular disease). It can also cause raised blood pressure.

Incidentally, some of the psychedelic drugs (see Chapter 5) are related to ergot.

The age of science

The entire pharmaceutical industry was initially founded on natural remedies. Until the 1830s the pharmacist's shop was a child's delight of rows of beautiful bottles and hundreds of mysterious drawers labelled with strange names such as Fol. Rosmarini (rosemary leaves), Ext. Rhubarb., Ext. Glycyrrh. (liquorice), Cinnamon bark, Tinct. Capsic. (cayenne Pepper), Tinct. Benz. Co., Senna Pod, Balsamum Peru., Gentian Violet, Tinct. Nux. Vom. (strychnine) and so on. These, and hundreds of other plant derivatives, were all claimed to be remedies and were compounded by the pharmacist on the spot into pills, infusions, tinctures and mixtures in accordance with an often elaborate prescription, written in Latin. Many of these prescriptions were virtually useless.

As the 19th century progressed chemists began increasingly to extract the active elements from medicinal plants. As a result, it was no longer necessary, in many cases, to depend on naturally occurring substances for drugs. Once the active ingredient had been identified, other related compounds could be chemically synthesized and tried. Yet even at the end of the 19th century, although doctors prescribed a wide range of drugs, there were only about a score of genuinely useful and effective drugs. These included opium for pain, digitalis for heart disease, quinine for malaria, atropine for eye diseases and abdominal colic, iodine for goitre, ether and chloroform anaesthetics, iron salts for anaemia, bicarbonate of soda for dyspepsia, salicylates for rheumatism and colchicum for gout.

In 1863 Louis Pasteur (1822-1895) demonstrated the existence of bacteria and in 1876 Robert Koch (1843-1910) cultivated the anthrax bacillus. These notable advances led to the production of vaccines for immunization. Pasteur developed vaccines against anthrax and rabies and Emil von Behring (1854-1917) developed an antitoxin against diphtheria in 1890. They also led to the search for drugs that could be taken internally to kill bacteria without killing the patient (see below).

Aspirin

The bark of some members of the willow family, the *Salinaceae*, has been known for centuries to have pain-relieving properties and to be useful in relieving rheumatism. One of the first formal reports on these properties appeared in 1763. Writing in the Philosophical Transactions of the Royal Society, the Reverend Edward Stone of Chipping Norton in Oxfordshire, England related '. . . there is a bark of an English tree which I have found by experience to be . . . very efficacious in curing agues and intermittent disorders. I have continued to use it for five years successively and successfully.'

Later, the active ingredient was found to be a substance called salicin and, from this, salicylic acid was derived and was widely used to relieve pain and reduce fever. The drug was especially useful in acute rheumatic fever. In 1853 Charles Gerhardt (1816-1856), the professor of chemistry at Strasbourg synthesized from it a new substance, acetyl salicylic acid. No one paid any attention to this substance at the time. Almost fifty years later, Heinrich Dreser (1860-1924) the Director of Research at the Bayer Pharmaceutical Company wondered if it would be possible to find a less irritating form of salicylic acid. One of his chemists remembered Gerhardt's compound and this was tested for irritation on the gills of live goldfish. Fortunately for mankind, the goldfish appear not to have objected too much for in 1899 the drug was given the trade name of Aspirin and made available to a grateful medical profession.

Aspirin was one of the first great commercial successes in the drug industry, and soon after the beginning of the 20th century the name of Bayer became famous around the world. Until recently Aspirin was, by far, the most widely used pain-relieving, fever-reducing, and anti-inflammatory drug. We now know that it has several other important actions – especially in its tendency to reduce the formation of blood clots – an action valuable in people liable to heart attacks. This and its other effects arise from its power to prevent the formation and release, by body cells, of powerful, pain-causing substances called prostaglandins.

Mercury drugs

Mercury has always fascinated people interested in magic and medicine. Both in its metallic form (quicksilver) and as various salts, especially mercurous chloride (calomel), mercury has been prescribed for almost every known disease – usually to the detriment of the patient. Mercury salts are highly poisonous, but this has not deterred intrepid physicians. A few of the more enlightened doctors, such as James Hamilton (1749-1833) who wrote a paper on the abuse of mercury in various diseases, were well aware of the dangers, but the majority continued to prescribe these remedies for all sorts of trivial conditions.

Until the 20th century, there was, however, one real justification for the use of mercury salts – they were the only thing known that could cure syphilis. In the doses needed to achieve this, the side effects were horrible. The teeth fell out, dribbling of saliva was constant, there was nausea, vomiting, diarrhoea, severe loss of weight and gross debility. Some patients went mad from the toxic effects on the brain; some just died. Familiarity with these effects was reflected in the grim humour of the often-quoted line '. . . a night with Venus and a lifetime with Mercury.' It was not until Paul Ehrlich (1854-1915) synthesized the organic arsenical compound Salvarsan in 1907 that mercury, as a drug for internal use, could at last be abandoned.

Ehrlich's discovery of Salvarsan

Paul Ehrlich knew that certain aniline dyes were ideal for staining bacteria. Clearly, the dyes had a particular affinity for the germs. This convinced him that it must be possible to find a safe drug that would latch on to particular germs present in the body and kill them. Jokingly, he called this drug his 'magic bullet'. So, quite logically, he decided to try certain organic compounds related to the dyes, but carrying a small quantity of the poison arsenic. These were called organic arsenicals. After testing hundreds of these compounds he found some that were so poisonous to certain organisms called trypanosomes that they would kill them in a dilution of one part in a million.

Ehrlich's research suggested that these organic compounds attached themselves to particular chemical groups in the organisms which he called 'chemoreceptors'. This was an entirely new idea at the time, but it was to become basic to future research on drugs.

Substance number 606 was synthesized but, for some reason, was not tried against trypanosomes. In 1909 a Japanese scientist called Sahachiro Hata, who was trying to find a safer cure for syphilis, came to Ehrlich's laboratory. By then Ehrlich had developed and tested about 3,000 compounds. To keep Sahachiro busy Ehrlich suggested that he should try all the organic arsenical compounds against the spirochaetes of syphilis. Compound 606 was found to be amazingly effective and was named 'Salvarsan'.

This was the 'magic bullet' Ehrlich had been seeking. Because of the chemoreceptors it could seek out the spirochaetes, wherever they were in the body, attach itself to them, and destroy them. This led to a greatly improved treatment for syphilis. When this sensational announcement was made in 1910 it was hard to decide which were louder – the cries of moral outrage over the realization that people could now get away with sin, or the demands for massive quantities of the drug from all over the world. Ehrlich's discovery prompted research which eventually flowered in the discovery of the sulpha drugs.

Drug developments in the 20th century

Paul Ehrlich's success started the search for further drugs that could kill germs without harming the patient. As late as the early 1930s it was generally believed that, although spirochaetes, trypanosomes and malarial parasites could be attacked by drugs such as the organic arsenicals, bacteria remained immune to such measures. In 1908 a young Austrian chemist, Paul Gelmo, working on textile dyes, synthesized the compound para-amino-benzene-sulphonamide. Gelmo wrote and published a paper about the new substance and then forgot about it.

The medical scientist Gerhard Domagk (1895-1964) tried many chemical substances against bacteria, among them the azo dyes which had long been used as bacterial stains for microscopy. In the course of his research he hit upon an azo compound, prontosil, that was closely related to Gelmo's compound. To his delight, prontosil was found to be not only wonderfully effective against streptococcal infections in mice, but also to be remarkably nontoxic to the mice.

At this point, Domagk's young daughter developed a severe streptococcal infection and 'blood poisoning' (septicemia) from a needle prick. Her life was in severe danger and, in despair, Domagk gave her a large dose of prontosil. Miraculously, the girl recovered completely. Soon it was soon discovered that it was not prontosil that was acting against the bacteria, but another substance, sulphanilamide, into which prontosil was being converted by the body. At once researchers started to try compounds of the sulphonamide group. This was the start of the sulphonamide revolution.

Thousands of related compounds were tried for their antimicrobial activity. In 1933 the drug company May and Baker marketed M&B 693 – sulphapyridine – with great success. This drug, the 693rd of the group to be tried, was used to treat the wartime Prime Minister Winston Churchill. Sulphathiazole was produced in 1940, sulphadimidine in 1941, and soon scores of other sulpha drugs rapidly appeared. These drugs saved countless lives in World War II. In 1942 it was discovered that a sulphonamide could stimulate insulin production from the pancreas. Sulpha derivatives, such as tolbutamide, are now universally used in late-onset diabetes. Sulphonamide research also led to the development of an important group of drugs that would increase the output of urine and relieve the body of unwanted water. These are called diuretic drugs.

Since the development of antibiotics, the use of the sulpha drugs has been limited, but they are still important and are widely used against streptococcal infections, urinary-tract infections and the serious inflammatory disease of the large intestine, ulcerative colitis.

The discovery of penicillin – the real story

It is one of the persistent fables of medicine that Alexander Fleming (1881-1955) discovered the antibiotic penicillin when a spore of *Penicillium notatum* mould floated in through the window of his laboratory in 1928, landed on a culture plate and destroyed some colonies of bacteria. Unfortunately, we now know that penicillin has to be present while the bacteria are reproducing to form colonies and would have no effect on colonies already formed. So this story must be discounted. It is almost certain that Fleming's plate had been contaminated before the bacteria grew, probably from a fungus laboratory on the floor below. There is also every reason to believe that the window by Fleming's bench was never opened. Culture plates are not left uncovered in well-conducted laboratories. It is more likely that Fleming misinterpreted what he saw on the plate and only dimly perceived that the new substance might have useful curative properties.

Fleming called the newly detected substance 'penicillin' and was able to show that it inhibited the growth of bacteria in low concentration, but was very unstable. The matter remained a laboratory curiosity and it was not until 1938 that Ernst Chain (1906-79), a refugee from Germany working with Professor Howard Florey (1898-1968) at Oxford University, England, became interested in Fleming's old reports and took up his work. Only then did the true significance of this wonderful substance begin to become clear. Chain and Florey were able to purify and obtain enough penicillin for human trials and the antibiotic era had begun.

Penicillin is produced by several moulds of the *Penicillium* and *Aspergillus* genera. Unlike anything ever used before to attack germs, it is almost completely non-poisonous to the body. Allergy to penicillin is common, but, that apart, it appears to be harmless. It was the first antibiotic successfully used internally to treat acute bacterial infections in humans.

Fleming shared the 1945 Nobel Prize for physiology or medicine with Chain and Florey.

Other drugs

The pace of drug development accelerated after the 1930s. During the 1940s and 1950s, thousands of valuable new drugs were developed and used successfully in the management of previously untreatable diseases. The first anticancer drugs appeared in the late 1940s, one of the earliest being developed from the World War I chemical weapon mustard gas. Largactil (chlorpromazine) – a break-through in the treatment of schizophrenia and other severe mental diseases, appeared in 1952 along with a number of antidepressant and tranquillizing drugs. The first corticosteroid drugs (steroids) were also introduced about this time.

Since the 1950s the pace of advance has been rapid. Newer and better anaesthetics, a wide range of anti-inflammatory and other corticosteroids, synthetic hormones, oral contraceptives, tranquillizers, anticoagulants, antiepilepsy drugs, antiviral drugs – the list is long. Millions of lives have been saved. Millions have been relieved of pain and distress. The happiness and the quality of life of millions has been enhanced.

The drug story goes on . . .

The story of levodopa

Back in 1914 the English physiologist Henry Dale (1875-1968) discovered a powerful substance in ergot called acetylcholine. When a tiny quantity of this substance was applied to nerve endings the associated muscles immediately contracted. Dale already suspected that a natural chemical substance was somehow involved in the transmission of nerve impulses at nerve-muscle junctions. Soon there was growing evidence that this substance was acetylcholine. By 1936 this was proved. Dale's work won him a Nobel prize but it was only the beginning of an enormous amount of research into the nature of these nerve activators, now called neurotransmitters.

In the course of time other neurotransmitters were found to be at work, not only in the peripheral nerves but also in the brain and spinal cord. Adrenaline, noradrenaline, serotonin, dopamine and many others were detected and their functions gradually understood. The greatest interest, of course, was in neurotransmitters acting within the brain itself. Research showed that the area of the brain richest in the neurotransmitter dopamine was a part called the substantia nigra, where dopamine is made. If the substantia nigra is stimulated naturally by nerve impulses, or artificially by electric currents, dopamine is released.

In the condition known as Parkinson's disease, or paralysis agitans, there is loss of substantia nigra cells, and the more severe the loss the more severe the disorder. As soon as these facts were known, attempts were made to give dopamine as a treatment. Unfortunately, dopamine does not pass from the blood into the brain and these attempts failed. In the late 1960s, however, it was found that the chemically related substance levodopa does pass easily from the blood to the brain and that this then converts to dopamine. When levodopa was tried in Parkinson's disease in 1969 at Beth Abraham Hospital in the Bronx, New York, the results were dramatic. 90% of those with Parkinson's disease responded, and experienced much less difficulty in moving and less rigidity and tremor. 30% appeared to have had an almost complete recovery. Unfortunately, we now know that in the course of a number of years the drug gradually loses its effect. Even so, levodopa provides an enormous improvement in the quality of life for people with Parkinsonism. Other drugs for the condition have also been developed.

The thalidomide story

In the autumn of 1961, doctors in West Germany realized that something very strange was happening. An epidemic of extraordinary malformations in babies was occurring. Some of these children had various internal abnormalities but most had the previously rare condition of phocomelia or 'seal limbs', in which the arms and legs were replaced by what looked like short flippers. The long bones of the limbs were absent or greatly shortened and the hands and feet, either virtually normal or rudimentary, were attached close to the body. In 1959, in West Germany, 17 cases had been seen. In 1960, 126. In 1961, 477 cases had occurred. Smaller outbreaks were reported from other countries.

No one could suggest a plausible explanation. All kinds of suggestions were made. Virus infections, radioactive fallout, X-rays, food preservatives, contraceptives were all considered, but none seemed likely to be the cause. The first really convincing evidence that a drug was the cause of these congenital defects came from the Australian obstetrician William McBride. The German paediatrician Widukind Lenz, of Hamburg University, also began to suspect that a drug might be the cause. Pregnant women who had been taking the sedative drug sold as Contergan, Distaval, Softenon, Kevadon, Talimol and under many other names had no suspicion that it might be dangerous. Indeed they often failed to mention the fact that they were taking it when completing research questionnaires.

One of the main selling points about Contergan had been its safety. When they were directly questioned, however, almost all the women who had had deformed babies were found to have taken the drug between the fourth and ninth weeks of pregnancy, when the fetus's limbs were developing. This drug was thalidomide.

In November 1961 the drug was withdrawn in West Germany and, in December 1961, it was withdrawn in Britain. The American paediatrician Helen Taussig, who was also investigating cases of phocomelia in Britain and Germany, also concluded that thalidomide was the cause. Her advice to the American Food and Drugs Administration (FDA) resulted in a refusal to licence the drug for the USA. In 1962 thalidomide was banned world-wide. Dr McBride was awarded a CBE, the Order of Australia and a gold medal from the French Institut de la Vie.

The full extent of the disaster did not become clear until the autumn of 1962. It was then admitted by the West German Public Health Ministry that since 1957, when – because of its safety – thalidomide had been approved for over-the-counter sale, it had caused about 10,000 cases of birth malformations in West Germany alone. About half of these babies had survived. In Britain, there were about 400 surviving malformed children. In Canada, more than 50, and in the USA only a handful. These had resulted from pre-marketing clinical trials. World-wide, there were estimated to be about 10,000 surviving deformed children. The drug had been sold under no fewer than 50 different trade names, many of them mixtures of thalidomide and other drugs – compounds such as Tensival, Valgraine, Valgis, Asmaval, Grippex, Peracon expectorans and Poltgripan. Even after the dangers of thalidomide were known by almost everyone, pregnant women were still taking the drug because they had no idea that it was in the preparation they were using. Everyone knew the name thalidomide, but this did not appear on any of the labels. The adverse publicity was more likely to refer to 'thalidomide' than to the many trade names.

The thalidomide tragedy wonderfully concentrated the minds of the pharmaceutical industry and of the various agencies respon-sible for licensing drugs. Up to this time, few had considered the possible effects of drugs on the early fetus and drugs were not routinely tested for such effects. Now the word 'teratogenicity' (the ability to cause serious developmental errors) was heard everywhere in drug circles. In Britain, the Committee on the Safety of Medicines was set up to monitor and control the production of new drugs. As a result, legislation was introduced to ensure that no new drug could be marketed until independent experts were agreed that it had been adequately tested and was safe. The committee was also concerned to ensure that doctors reported adverse reactions to drugs. The American Food and Drugs Administration (FDA), set up after a poisonous sulpha preparation had been released in 1937, killing 107 people, was already performing this function. Where such drug regulatory authorities did not exist, they were set up all over the world.

There is a sad postscript to the thalidomide story. Dr William McBride seemed to be impelled to try to repeat the triumph that had made him world-famous in 1961. He began to issue warnings about other drugs, such as imipramine and dicyclomine-doxylamine (Debendox), claiming that these drugs were also the cause of fetal abnormalities. When his claims extended to the sedative scopolamine hydrobromide, widely used in anaesthesia, investigation showed that he had been falsifying the results of his experiments. His earlier claims of the dangers of other drugs were also discredited. In August 1993 Dr McBride's name was struck off the Medical Register. He had been found guilty of scientific fraud.

Tailor-made drugs

Once the receptor theory of drug action was well established, research went ahead rapidly. Studies of the actions of the hormone noradrenaline, for instance, showed that it acted through a group of chemical receptors, on the surface of cells, called adrenergic receptors. These were not all the same. There were two classes, alpha and beta receptors. Receptors could be stimulated by noradrenaline or by similar substances. Thus adrenaline, acting on beta receptors in the heart, increased the rate and force of contraction.

It had been known for many years that the ergot alkaloids could cause tight constriction of arteries and it now became apparent that these were acting at the alpha adrenergic receptor sites. The work of

Dale on ergot effects as early as 1906 had thrown much light on this. These important facts indicated that if chemicals could be found to block these receptor sites, thus reducing the action of noradrenaline, these would enable us to control the often adverse effects of the hormone.

Such ideas formed the basis for the eventual production of a wide range of valuable drugs – drugs that had the same general chemical shape as adrenaline, so that they would fit into the receptors, but would be subtly different so that they would not trigger off the normal effect. The first of these blocker drugs – known as 'beta-blockers' because they block the beta-adrenergic receptors – was propranolol (trade names Berkolol, Inderal). This drug fits into the beta receptors and blocks them so that noradrenaline cannot stimulate them. As a result the heart rate is slowed, angina pectoris is relieved and high blood pressure is reduced. It can, however, cause the air tubes to tighten and so may provoke asthma. Many other beta-blocking drugs with highly selective actions have been developed. They are all antagonistic to adrenaline and so are generally calming in their effects.

The development of propranolol in 1958 was the work of a remarkable man, James Whyte Black (1924-   ), now Sir James, who was, at the time, senior pharmacologist at ICI. Black was well aware of the receptor theory and had the chemical know-how to create the appropriate new chemical compound. Later, when he was at the pharmaceutical laboratory of Smith Kline and French, Black scored another brilliant receptor first when he produced a chemical that would compete with histamine for access to the H-2 histamine receptors in the stomach (see below).

Receptor blockade was obviously a winner and scientists started to look more widely. They knew that certain cells in the body, stimulated in a particular way, release the powerful substance histamine into the surrounding tissues. Histamine is very nasty stuff and causes flushing, itching, skin weals, shock, allergy, and asthma. It also stimulates the secretion of acid in the stomach.

The first drugs able to block the action of histamine were discovered in 1937, but it was not until 1944 that a practical and safe antihistamine drug was developed. This was followed by a flood of similar drugs. Unfortunately, although very useful, none of these drugs had any action on the stomach acid secreting effect of histamine. It was a long time before the researchers discovered that there were two kinds of histamine receptors – H1 receptors and H2 receptors. Antihistamines were H1 blockers. No H2 blockers were known.

More than 30 years were to pass before drugs were developed that selectively blocked the action of histamine in producing stomach acid – the H2 blockers. Like other blocking drugs, these substances act by occupying the receptor sites and preventing the activating substance, in this case histamine, from working. What scientists, especially James Black, did was to take a histamine molecule and deliberately try to alter it so that it would still fit into the receptors but would be unable to trigger off the usual effect. About 200 attempts were made before, in 1972, Black and his team produced an effective drug. This drug worked very well, but to their great disappointment it was found to damage white blood cell production and had to be withdrawn.

Fortunately, a small modification solved the problem and resulted in the drug cimetidine (Tagamet, Algitec, Dyspamet, Galenamet). Soon a closely related drug ranitidine (Zantac) was produced. Cimetidine and ranitidine changed the whole management of conditions such as stomach and duodenal ulcers (localized partial destruction of the lining), caused by excessive production of stomach acid. It reduced both the volume and the acidity of the acid produced and it reduced the production of the digestive enzyme pepsin which, in peptic ulceration, digests the stomach or duodenal wall. The clinical effects were excellent and profits from Zantac soon rose higher than those from any other drug in production.

James Black was knighted in 1981 and was awarded the Nobel Prize for physiology or medicine in 1988.

Drugs by genetic engineering

Genetic engineering is the technology of deliberate alteration of the genetic material DNA (deoxyribonucleic acid). This is done by using one or more of a large number of chemical activators (enzymes), each of which can cut DNA at a particular known place.

Cut DNA has 'sticky' ends, and if a suitable length of DNA from somewhere else is put into the living cell, it will glue itself into the gap. The cell now has new genetics, and all the cells that arise from it will be identical. The enzymes that cut DNA are called 'restriction enzymes'.

Under suitable conditions, one bacterium, such as an *E. coli*, divides into two full-size germs in about half an hour. By the end of the hour there are four. By the end of the second hour there are 16. A population that doubles every half hour increases, in the absence of losses, to about 5000 million million million million individuals in one day. All these individuals have identical genes, and the population is called a clone. Suppose the first one had had its DNA altered. It might, for instance, have had the gene that programs for the protein human insulin inserted. In a few days the large clone grown from this bacterium in a fermentation would produce a great deal of human insulin. This is how insulin, needed to treat the disease diabetes, is now made. Unlike the ox or pig insulin previously used, human insulin does not cause the diabetics who need it to produce dangerous antibodies.

Genetic engineering methods are being used to produce a range of valuable drugs. These include growth hormone, antigrowth hormone and the natural antivirus substance interferon. Another important advance is the production of tissue plasminogen activator (TPA). This substance, given soon after a heart attack, can dissolve the clot that is blocking a coronary artery and restore full function of the heart. There is no theoretical reason why the whole range of human hormones, together with many other naturally-produced substances of medical importance, should not be made in this way.

Genetically engineered vaccines are also being enthusiastically researched. Scientists have discovered that they can use restriction enzymes to remove from viruses or bacteria the genes that make them dangerous. Clones from these safe organisms make excellent vaccines. The cloned organisms can no longer cause disease, but they still stimulate the body to make antibodies to repel the natural organisms.

2. HOW NEW DRUGS ARE MADE AND TESTED

The discovery, development, testing and successful marketing of a new drug is a very complicated, expensive and slow business. Indeed, the wonder is that any new drugs ever do get produced. Fortunately for suffering mankind the profit motive tends to overcome such obstacles. A really successful drug, like Zantac or Zovirax, generates enormous profits. On the day this was written, the financial pages featured a 45½p rise in Glaxo shares because, the day before, the American Food and Drugs Administration (FDA) had given approval for the general marketing in the USA of the antinausea drug Zofran. Since February 1991 the drug has been available for use by people on anticancer therapy. Now it has access to the much wider post-operative sickness market. Note how popular the initial letter Z has become for new trade names. Whatever the reason for this, it has nothing to do with chemical terminology.

A new drug now often takes some 20 years to be carried through to full production, and even to reach production is the exception rather than the rule. Some estimates have it that only one suggested drug in 10,000 gets as far as testing on humans, and less than one in 100 of those taken seriously and tested eventually become licensed drugs. The great majority are abandoned at an early stage.

Producing new drugs

There are several ways of starting to produce a new drug. Prior to the development of modern biochemical science we had to rely on the discovery of new plants or inorganic compounds with pharmacological properties. Although there are still plenty of pharmacologically-active plants to be tried, this method is now rare. Today, much of the research into the production of new drugs starts with the knowledge of the action of natural body substances, especially those such as hormones and nerve stimulators (neurotransmitters) that bring about a change in the body. Once these substances have been identified and their chemical composition established, it usually becomes possible to synthesize them and then to try out various minor modifications of the molecule to see whether a worthwhile drug results. A great deal of work is also done in modifying existing drugs in the hope of making them more efficacious, or safer, or both.

Chemists can now turn out entirely new substances in enormous numbers. A knowledge of the chemical structure and of the general effects on the body of various molecules provides an indication that some of these new substances might have medically useful effects. So thousands of them are tried, using very sophisticated methods. Most are dropped either because they have no effect at all, or because the effect is undesired or useless, or because they are too poisonous. Only a tiny minority offer a hint of possible value. Those that do may then be further modified chemically to try to enhance the effect.

All this makes drug research sound like a hit-and-miss affair, but this is only one of the ways in which new drugs are found. In research to discover a new drug to fight a particular kind of cancer, for instance, there is simply no question of just trying one thing after another in the hope that one might work. Anticancer drugs, like all other major classes of drugs, have to be based on a detailed knowledge of the nature of the disease process. Scientists hoping to improve the outlook for patients with cancer can never know enough about what happens in cells when they undergo cancerous change. In fact, the amount that is known about the mechanisms of cancer is quite extraordinary and fills hundreds of books. Almost all the work currently in progress in the development of anticancer drugs is based on this ever-extending knowledge.

Drug toxicity

Once a new drug has been shown to have valuable properties, decisions have to be made about how poisonous (toxic) it is. Every drug is toxic; the question is, how much of a margin is there between the dose that produces the desired effect and the dose that poisons or kills the patient. The difference between the two levels is known as the therapeutic index. This is, in theory, the largest dose that can be tolerated divided by the smallest dose that cures. Scientists don't actually do this sum, but they recognize very clearly that a drug with a high therapeutic index is a safe drug and one with a low index is dangerous. Even so, especially in the case of anticancer drugs, it is often necessary, for want of anything better, to use drugs with a low therapeutic index. The ideal drug, of course, would have an infinite therapeutic index. Unfortunately, even pure water is toxic if you get enough of it. A few drugs have a remarkably high therapeutic index. Allergy aside, penicillin, for instance, can safely be given in dosages thousands of times greater than those necessary to cure infections. Unfortunately, it is rare for drugs to have such a high therapeutic index. Most highly active drugs must be given in carefully regulated doses.

Toxicity testing, which includes checks whether drugs might cause fetal abnormalities, must be done on mice or other small animals. Various levels of dosage are given, starting with very small doses, and the outcome is compared with a control group of closely similar animals who are not given the drug. There is, unfortunately, no other way of finding out whether potentially important drugs can safely be tried out on humans. As well as checking for toxic effects, researchers are, of course, interested in the degree to which the desired effect of the drug is achieved.

Concerns about cancer

One of the many concerns of the drug developers is whether the drug itself, whatever its purpose, can cause cancer. This is not such a straightforward concern, or such an easy matter, as might be imagined. We now know, for instance, that quite a number of cancers that can occur in people in the latter part of life are caused by exposure to various chemical substances many years before. Most of these have been traced to industrial chemicals to which workers were exposed in the course of their employment and there is now a fairly long list of these carcinogens, as they are called. This observation is worrying, as it would seem to imply that no drug can be considered safe until trials have shown that it does not cause cancer up to 30 or 40 years after it has been used. This would seem to put a real damper on drug research.

At the same time, however, knowledge of this kind has helped scientists to get a very useful idea of the kind of compounds that are liable to cause cancerous changes in cells. They also understand very much more clearly than ever before, exactly how these chemicals cause the DNA changes that lead to cancer. Obviously, research workers are going to be particularly careful if any drugs they are investigating resemble known carcinogens, either in their chemical structure or in their effect. Many drugs used in medicine fall into this category.

Understandable emotional attitudes about carcinogenicity in drugs has led to odd situations. Earlier this century the US Government passed laws to the effect that no substance known to be capable of causing cancer, *however much of it was taken*, could be included in a food or a drug. At first sight, this seems sensible. It didn't, however, quite work out that way. Scientists were soon advising the government that a huge number of substances were capable of causing cancer if a large enough dose were given. These included many substances that almost everyone was eating. Even nickels and dimes proved carcinogenic, and the authors of one report to the government ironically recommended that the legislature should consider banning money as unsafe. Compliance with the law would mean that many substances of great economic importance would have to be outlawed. It was not long before the regulations were amended.

Human trials

Once a drug is shown to be free from obvious toxic effects, the time has come for properly conducted trials on humans. While there is a close correlation between the effects of most drugs on animals and their effects on humans, this cannot be assumed always to be true. Usually, a drug that does not work on small animals will not work on humans either. Such a drug would immediately be abandoned. Sometimes, a drug that works well on animals will not work at all on humans. In this case, attempts might be made to modify the molecule. And just occasionally, a drug that does not work on animals will work well on humans.

People who are asked to volunteer for new drug trials must be made clearly aware of what is happening. When they give written consent, it must be *informed* consent – they must fully appreciate the risks. Initial testing is done on very small groups of people, perhaps no more than half a dozen, certainly less than 100, who are often volunteers from the staff of the laboratory carrying out the research. Medical students often volunteer for these trials. These people must be in excellent health and will be carefully examined before the trial. Half of them are used as controls and the other half are given a single dose of the drug in the smallest amount estimated to produce some effect. This dose is based on the results of the animal trials. These preliminary trials are done under careful medical supervision.

Over the course of several weeks, alternative groups acting as controls and subjects, are given gradually increasing doses of the drug. Appropriate tests, such as measurements of various blood changes, are carried out and checked before each change in the dosage. Most cases involve taking large numbers of blood samples. As a result of these preliminary trials it is usually possible to determine:

- an appropriate dose for the drug
- the dose range that can be tolerated
- whether the drug is readily absorbed from the intestine
- the rate at which it is excreted from the body
- how toxic it is
- which organ or organs are affected by any toxic effect
- whether the drug shows the desired therapeutic action

In the second phase of testing, larger numbers of volunteers are used – often several hundred. There is never any question of a drug being tried on people who are unaware of what is going on. All are volunteers who have agreed in writing to take part. The people involved in this stage are, however, people suffering from the condition the drug is aimed to treat. The trial will often be conducted in hospital. The aims of this stage are to assess the clinical usefulness of the drug and to find out what side effects are caused and how severe they are. A drug may have to be abandoned at this stage either for lack of efficacy or lack of safety, or both.

In the third phase of testing, much larger numbers of volunteers, sometimes several thousands, are involved. Such third stage trials are usually conducted simultaneously in many hospitals. The main object, at this stage, is to find out whether the drug offers any substantial advantage over existing drugs used for the condition concerned and to acquire statistical data on unwanted reactions.

None of all this can legally happen without official knowledge, registration and regulation. Different countries have different regulatory arrangements, some more stringent than others. These official bodies have to be kept informed, at every stage, of what is going on. In some cases a clinical trial certificate, giving permission to proceed, must be obtained. In the USA, the regulations administered by the Food and Drug Administration (FDA) are particularly strict. Before a new drug can be licensed regulatory authorities usually have to be sent an enormous amount of information – often hundreds of large boxes of data. This comprises detailed descriptions of every stage of the work, from the very beginning.

Double-blind trials

A double-blind trial is a way of organizing the assessment of a drug or a new medical treatment, in which neither the patient nor the persons conducting the trial know which one of two identical-seeming treatments is genuine and which is a dummy. In the case of a trial of a new drug, a pharmacist makes up two sets of tablets or capsules that cannot be distinguished by appearance, taste, etc. One set contains the active ingredient and the other an inert (inactive) substance. Only the pharmacist knows which is which. The medication is allocated randomly and the key as to who gets what is locked away until the end of the trial. After the results are known, the key is checked to see whether those who had the active drug did significantly better than those who took the dummy.

The purpose of double-blindness is to balance out the placebo effect which is so powerful that a single trial of a drug, of no actual medical value, will often show an apparently useful effect. The placebo effect is a tendency for a person taking a remedy, or a supposed remedy, to feel better even if the treatment has no actual medical value.

Publication

Third-phase trials are usually conducted by hospital doctors and when these are complete the results are often published in medical journals, under the authorship of the doctors concerned. A significant proportion of the output of many medical journals is devoted to the results of new drug trials. This is a handy way of getting into print – something that most hospital doctors are interested in.

Publications of this kind do, however, serve several useful purposes. They attract the critical attention of other doctors who will not hesitate to write in to point out inadequacies in the design of the trial, fallacies in the reasoning or errors in the statistics. They encourage doctors to cooperate closely with the pharmaceutical manufacturers, and they draw detailed attention to valuable new drugs so that doctors can improve the treatment of their patients.

Formulation

Long before a drug reaches third-phase trials a lot of work will have been put into finding out the best way to present the drug for human use. This is called formulation. Essentially it is a matter of selecting the best inert substances with which to mix the drug so that it can be presented as tablets, capsules or solutions for injection. These non-drug substances, or excipients, may be binding agents, disintegrating or distributing agents, lubricants or simple fillers. The actual weight of active substance of a drug required for a single dose varies enormously, from millionths of a gram (micrograms) to several grams. Most drugs require to be taken in a dose of tens or hundreds of milligrams (thousandths of a gram). This means that drugs usually have to be considerably diluted to make up the normal bulk for a tablet or capsule.

There are dozens of different ways in which a new drug can be formulated. In many cases the basic formulation is determined by the nature of the active substance – whether solid or liquid, for instance. Apart from tablets and capsules, drugs may be formulated in many different ways. These include:

- liquid-containing gelatine capsules
- liquid-containing glass vials
- solid powders in vials packaged with a separate liquid
- ointments
- creams
- lotions
- eye and ear drops
- rectal suppositories
- vaginal pessaries or tampons

- skin patches
- implantable slow-release tablets

Tablets can be made in various shapes and sizes and can be scored with a deep 'break-bar' for easy division into two. Some tablets are layered. In general, tablets are made simply by compressing the mixture of ingredients together in a mould. Tablets are then film-coated to provide a protective surface layer that increases their strength, prevents crumbling or chipping, reduces the effects of moisture and light and may even help to mask a bitter or unpleasant taste. The film coating can be coloured, if desired. While it is important that tablets should be physically stable to resist damage during manufacture and bulk packaging, it is equally important that they should not be so stable that they do not break up or dissolve after being swallowed. Irritating, unduly stable tablets, such as non-soluble Aspirin can be dangerous and can cause stomach ulceration.

An unusual tablet shape can help to establish the identity of a particular product and may improve popularity. Capsule colouring is also a help in product identification. Capsules may be of various combinations of two colours – one for each half – or may be banded. Some contain the drug as a fine powder, some as granules. The latter may be of several different rates of solution to provide a timed-release effect. Granular formulation also allows a combination of different drugs to be given together. Manufacturers are also aware that the acceptability of a drug depends, to a degree, on the appearance of the formulation. If a drug is for any reason unattractive, patients may not take it.

Packaging

The actual packaging of drugs is determined, to some extent, by the need to protect them against light and high humidity. Some drugs lose their activity if exposed to moisture and high temperatures. Some even become more toxic. Such considerations might decree that drugs are packaged in sealed glass bottles, coloured to keep out white light. In other cases, plastic bottles, individual dose blister packs (unit packaging) or sealed paper or plastic strips may be more appropriate. The choice of plastic may be important. Some drugs, for instance, interact with polystyrene. Decisions also have to be made about the design of containers. There are pressures on manufacturers to package drugs in child-proof bottles, such as those in which the lid cannot be removed unless it is turned to a certain position. Sometimes these bottles prove too difficult to open, especially by the elderly and infirm, or by those with arthritis or poor vision.

In spite of optimum packaging, many drugs cannot be relied on to retain their full potency or safety indefinitely. For these and other reasons, most drugs are given a definite shelf life, after which they should not be used. The determination of an appropriate shelf life is not particularly easy and various forms of accelerated storage tests are used.

Sorting out the problems of packaging for bulk production may be very expensive and may take many months.

Marketing

Doctors are often not particularly sympathetic towards the marketing activities of drug manufacturers. This is partly because doctors are individualists who like to make up their own minds about what to prescribe, and tend to resent any suspicion that they are being pressured into using a particular product. So manufacturers representatives often find themselves sitting for long hours in doctors' waiting rooms, nursing large briefcases full of samples.

From the manufacturer's point of view the matter is quite different. The marketing department is vital to the commercial success of the whole business and must be involved in every new product almost from the beginning. People on the research and development side cannot be expected to take a realistically commercial view of the business and tend to get carried away by their interest in applied science. They might, for instance, propose a drug that the marketing people know would be impossible to sell. They might suggest getting into a sector of the market that is already heavily covered by the products of competitors. They might suggest a timing for a new product that could prejudice the success of the whole venture.

Marketing has become highly specialized, even to the extent that there are different marketing groups for the different classes of drugs (see Chapter 3). The members of these groups become very knowledgeable about their particular drug category and work in close association with the relevant scientific specialists. They know the market for their own class of pharmaceuticals, they know the leading medical figures in their particular line, and they know what is likely to be commercially successful. They are well aware that, however skilful the marketing, a drug is not going to sell if it offers no convincing advantage over a dozen existing medications in the field.

The marketing department is, of course, deeply involved in advertising. This has many aspects. Huge amounts of money are spent in advertising new products to the medical profession, mainly, but not exclusively, by advertisements in medical newspapers and many of the medical journals. The principal journals, such as *The Lancet*, the *British Medical Journal* (BMJ), or the *New England Journal of Medicine*, either do not accept drug advertising or do so to a very limited extent. Less prestigious journals often carry such heavy drug advertising that it sometimes seems hard to find the real text.

Marketing personnel aim to build up good relations with doctors. This is achieved not so much by crude methods of free gifts of ballpoint pens, subsidised lunches and flights to medical conferences in exotic places, as by the provision of real information on new products. One important part of this involves the production of properly prepared product brochures, monographs and even books. Some of the foremost manufacturers produce excellent specialist texts of the highest quality on all sorts of subjects. Some even provide postgraduate medical educational facilities in the form of medical museums and multimedia educational products.

It is common for hospital clinical tutors, concerned with postgraduate medical education and continuing nurse training to have excellent relationships with many manufacturer's representatives. These assist in the organization of clinical meetings by providing medical films, video shows, and lectures and demonstrations of new products. Often the subject of the meeting will have nothing to do with any of the manufacturers' products, and the representatives will be content if they are allowed to set up a small promotional stand with product literature and samples.

How drugs are named

This is a major concern of the manufacturers who know that, other things being equal, a name can make or mar a new product. Names not only identify a drug, they also create an image. Zantac is a good drug, but it did it no harm to be named in such a way as to remind everyone that it is an antacid (a drug to reduce the acidity in the stomach). With this drug, Glaxo also broke the long-standing rule that it was a good idea to choose names at the beginning of the alphabet so that the drug would appear near the top of lists of drug names. Actually, Zantac's phenomenal commercial success has led to an increasing vogue for names beginning with Z.

Once a new trade name has been selected, it can be registered and the company can sue anyone else who uses it commercially. This introduces another difficulty in that a very thorough search has to be made to ensure that the proposed new name has not already been registered, not just for a drug, but for *anything*. This is one reason why new drug names often sound rather odd. There are certain basic rules that manufacturers try to follow in choosing names. They must remember that a name that is perfectly acceptable in the home country might be offensive or ridiculous in another country. Names must not only be unique, but they must also be unlikely to be confused with any other existing drug name. They should be short, easy to pronounce, as similar as possible to the generic name (see below), and should, if possible, suggest the action of the drug. Many manufacturers incorporate the name of the firm into the drug name. Some, like ICI with its beta blockers, go in for anagrams (Inderal, Alderin, Eraldin).

Finally, to make matters worse, manufacturers have to choose three names – the chemical name, the generic name and the trade name. Chemical names are usually allocated by the chemists and no one cares if they take up two lines of print. Only chemists are going to be interested. Generic names (see page 148) have to follow certain rules laid down by various international and national committees. These, and other restrictions have made the job so difficult that many new names are now, in fact, generated by computers that simply invent and print out all possible names conforming to these rules. These lists are then considered by naming committees. That is when the real problems start.

3. THE MAIN DRUG GROUPS

When doctors talk about drugs, they don't usually mean narcotics or recreational drugs. They mean any substance that can be introduced into the body, by any route, to bring about some change. Drugs even include substances used to help in finding out what is wrong with you, but, of course, most drugs are used to help cure or relieve disease. Today, there remains almost no disease for which there is no drug useful treatment.

Drugs have many uses. The most important of these are:

- to regularize and control abnormal conditions of body and mind
- to replace missing substances
- to kill viruses, bacteria, fungi and other damaging organisms
- to suppress or modify some aspect of normal body function
- to relieve pain or discomfort

Most of the really important drugs are available only on a doctor's prescription and, in some cases, strict regulations apply to the way in which they are prescribed. You can buy non-prescription, or 'over-the-counter' drugs without restriction in a chemist's shop. They are, in general, reasonably safe even if you take a little more than the recommended dose. But you should remember that *any* drug, however seemingly innocuous, can be dangerous if taken in large excess.

This chapter is primarily about the different classes of drugs, rather than about diseases and other medical conditions. But the whole point about drugs is that they are used to correct these conditions, so quite a lot must be said about the conditions that drugs can cure. Don't get the idea that medical treatment is a simple matter of knee-jerk prescription of drugs on the 'This patient can't sleep; she needs Mogadon.' basis. This kind of thing does happen, but it is bad medicine. So, mixed up with the facts about the drug groups and how they are used to treat disease, you will find a lot of useful medical advice thrown in. To help you to find the condition you may be interested in, there are plenty of cross-references to guide you from the conditions to the relevant drug groups.

Drug side effects

People taking prescription drugs are rightly concerned about side effects, so you will find plenty about these, also, in this chapter. A side effect is any action not intended, and there are many of these. Different drugs may cause different side effects and these include nausea, vomiting, loss of appetite, diarrhoea, constipation, drowsiness, tiredness, a dry mouth, blurring of vision, a rapid heartbeat, difficulty in urinating, even impotence. Some drugs can lower the blood pressure and cause fainting. Others may upset the menstrual cycle.

Drugs that act on the nervous system, such as sedatives, narcotics and tranquillizers, can affect mood, judgment, memory and motivation – usually for the worse. These drugs may even disturb coordination and affect balance.

Drug allergy is not, strictly, a side effect, but people who suffer allergic reactions to drugs might consider the distinction academic. Allergy may feature a skin rash, itching, raised purplish skin swellings, asthma, tummy upset, fainting, shock or collapse. Drug allergy is especially dangerous when the drug concerned is given by injection, so doctors are always wary of this. Usually they give a very small test dose at first and then, after a few minutes, if nothing untoward has happened, the full dose.

Allergic reactions do not occur the first time a drug is given. The sensitivity has to be acquired from previous contact, but you can get an allergic reaction from a drug with a completely different name from the one you are allergic to, if it happens to belong to the same group, or even to be identical. This is one of the many disadvantages of the present chaotic system of naming drugs (see Chapter 7).

Poisoning

Poisoning by drugs is surprisingly common, and generally means that too much of the drug has accumulated in the body. This may be because too much has been given or because, although the dosage was normal, the rate of loss of the drug, by breakdown or excretion, is reduced. Kidney disease, for instance, commonly prevents drugs being lost from the body at a normal rate.

The liver is especially liable to be poisoned. This is because most drugs get to the liver in high concentrations. Hepatitis, even death of liver cells (liver atrophy) and liver failure, can be caused by drugs. The kidneys, too, in attempting to get rid of drugs, may be exposed to toxic levels. In the days of the sulphonamides, these drugs sometimes occurred in such high concentrations in the kidneys that they formed crystals that blocked and damaged the tubules. Drugs can cause blindness, by damaging the retinas or optic nerves, and deafness, by affecting the sensitive hair cells in the cochlea of the inner ear.

The thalidomide disaster (see Chapter 1) alerted everyone to the high degree of sensitivity of the young fetus to any possibly damaging influence that can get to it. As a result, doctors are rightly very cautious when prescribing for women in early pregnancy.

Many drugs are habit-forming and this must be balanced against their advantages. 'Sleeping pills' and 'sedatives', once widely and freely prescribed, are now used with much greater caution. This applies to drugs such as the benzodiazepines (e.g. Mogadon, Valium, Librium) and the barbiturates. Other habit-forming drugs prescribed with caution include opiate drugs such as morphine, the amphetamines, cocaine, and the wide range of powerful painkillers such as methadone. Accidental or suicidal poisoning from drugs is very common and child-proof packaging methods are now standard. Some drugs commonly used in suicide attempts, such as paracetamol (Panadol) are being combined with an antidote.

Drug interactions

Unfortunately, many people have to take more than one drug at a time, and, even more regrettably, drugs are sometimes prescribed without adequate knowledge of what the patient is already taking. Drug interactions are the adverse effects that can occur when separate drugs are taken simultaneously, and the drugs act on each other in such a way as to increase the toxicity or reduce the effectiveness of one or both. Drug interactions may be dangerous.

The commonest interaction is well known – the additive effect of similar drugs or of drugs having similar actions – and the commonest example is the additive effect of alcohol on any of the sedatives or tranquillizers. This can lead to a dangerous degree of sedation, and may, for instance, make driving hazardous. The law does not excuse a transgressor simply because is was a drug, rather than drink, that led to the crime.

Sometimes drugs combine to reduce the effect of both. One drug may interfere with the absorption of another. Drugs are commonly bound to, and carried by, proteins in the blood. One drug can sometimes displace another from its bound form, releasing it so that its action is stronger. Much of what happens in cells is controlled by thousands of different chemical activators called enzymes. Drugs can interfere with enzyme action, either enhancing or interfering with it. Drugs are often broken down by enzymes, so that they do not act for so long. Some other drugs, by interfering with the breaking-down enzymes, allow the first drug to act for much longer than normal. Some drugs prevent the action of others by blocking the receptor sites on cell membranes where many drugs act.

Drugs and elderly people

Elderly people have far more trouble from prescribed drugs than younger people. Often without knowing it, they suffer adverse effects directly attributable to the medication they are taking. Every time this problem has been investigated, alarming facts have come to light – people being seriously overdosed, people taking drugs which react dangerously with one another, people taking medicines whose actions cancel one another, and so on. Often more than one doctor is involved, and sometimes each is unaware of what the other has been prescribing. It is not particularly uncommon for doctors to diagnose senile dementia or Alzheimer's disease, when, in fact, the trouble is due to overtreatment with sedatives or other drugs.

Elderly people tend to have faith in medicines and will often buy additional remedies from a chemist's or even take medicines recommended and given to them by their friends from well-stocked bathroom cabinets. Some herbal remedies contain active and potentially harmful ingredients and overuse of these can add to the problem. They may even interact with prescribed medication.

The elderly often have more than one disorder, so multiple prescribing is common. There may be tablets for the heart; tablets for blood pressure; tablets to help with sleeping and tablets to keep the arthritic pain under control; tablets to get rid of the swelling of the ankles and the fluid in the lungs, and tablets to stop the urine from burning. More than four separate remedies should be exceptional, but there are plenty of people taking ten.

If you are in this sort of situation, you are entitled to try to make sure that you are not being harmed. It is a good idea to write down the name of everything you are taking and how many per day. If possible, put down what you think the medication is for. Write down any herbal or nonprescription medicine you are taking. Don't miss anything out just because you have been taking it for years. Write down, also, any symptoms or effects you have had since starting any of the medicines. Then take your list to your doctor and ask him or her to check it. You are quite likely to find that several drugs will be struck off the list. It is perfectly proper for you to ask your doctor whether all these medicines are really necessary, whether any of the symptoms you are having may be caused by the treatment and whether any of the drugs have been prescribed to treat the side effects of others. This is sometimes unavoidable but is often just the result of hasty medical management. In such cases, you are entitled to expect your doctor to think again.

THE A TO Z OF DRUG ACTIONS, USES AND SIDE EFFECTS

Most of the names of the drug groups will probably be unfamiliar to you. To try to get round this problem, however, many of the conditions for which drugs are used are included among the headings. You may not know, for instance, what angiotensin converting enzyme inhibitors are. But if it is high blood pressure you are interested in, and you look up high blood pressure, you will be referred to this useful group of drugs, as well as to others. It is also worth looking through the headings starting with 'anti-', as many of the conditions you might be concerned with will be found there. Because much of medicine is concerned with attacking disease, the word 'anti-' appears often.

Many drugs are mentioned in this chapter. Names with capital initial letters are trade names; those with lower-case initial letters are the official or generic names. In many cases the generic name is given first, followed by a common trade name in brackets. Regrettably, there are so many different trade names for many generic drugs that only a selection can be given. Check Chapter 7 for information on generic and trade names. Note also that words in small capital letters are cross references to entries in this chapter.

ACE inhibitors

See ANGIOTENSIN CONVERTING ENZYME INHIBITORS.

Acne

See RETINOID DRUGS.

Acromegaly

See DOPAMINE RECEPTOR AGONISTS.

Adrenaline-like drugs

See ADRENORECEPTOR AGONISTS, SYMPATHOMIMETIC DRUGS.

Adrenoreceptor agonists

An agonist is something that causes an action, usually an action similar to that of a natural body substance. Adrenoreceptor agonists are drugs with the same action as adrenaline – the natural body 'fright, fight or flight' hormone. These drugs are often very useful and can, occasionally, be life-saving. They have several effects. They can:

- widen air tubes (bronchi) tightly narrowed in asthma
- control severe allergic reactions
- reverse certain cases of acute heart failure
- prevent premature labour

- control certain kinds of glaucoma (excess internal eye pressure)
- narrow skin blood vessels to prolong the action of local anaesthetics

Air tube widening drugs include salbutamol (Ventolin) and salmeterol (Serevent). Adrenaline itself is used in dangerous allergic reactions and to prolong the effect of local anaesthetic injections. Adrenaline drops (Eppy) are used in treating chronic simple glaucoma – the common type mainly affecting elderly, people. Heart failure may be treated with dobutamine (Dobutrex), and premature labour with salbutamol or ritodrine.

The side effects are those that might be expected from adrenaline – jumpiness, shakiness, tremor, restlessness, anxiety, a fast pulse, a rise in blood pressure, even attacks of angina. Such effects are very rare when these drugs are used by inhalation or in eye drops or local anaesthetics.

Adrenoreceptor blockers

These are drugs that prevent adrenaline from acting in various ways. In general, their action is the opposite of that of the adrenoreceptor agonists (see above). They are used to relax arteries and thus lower very high blood pressure and to relieve the strain on the heart in conditions of heart failure. They include prazosin (Hypovase), doxazosin (Cardura) and indoramin (Baratol). Overdosage causes a severe drop in blood pressure, a slow pulse, nausea, vomiting and diarrhoea, a dry mouth, flushed skin, convulsions, drowsiness and coma.

Agonist

Any foreign substance that acts at a cell receptor site to produce the same, or a similar, effect as the normal body's chemical messenger. Many drugs are physiological agonists.

Allergic rhinitis

See ANTIHISTAMINE DRUGS.

Allergy

See ANTIHISTAMINE DRUGS.

Alpha blocker drugs

Also called alpha-ADRENOCEPTOR BLOCKERS. These are drugs that cause widening of arteries (vasodilatation) by blocking the action of adrenaline-like hormones. They include tolazoline, indoramin, phenoxybenzamine and thymoxamine. Overdosage causes a severe drop in blood pressure, a fast pulse, nausea, vomiting and diarrhoea, a dry mouth, flushed skin, convulsions, drowsiness and coma.

Aminoglycoside antibiotic drugs

See ANTIBIOTIC DRUGS.

Amoebic dysentery

See ANTI-AMOEBIC DRUGS.

Amphetamine drugs

A class of drugs formerly used widely for appetite control and to treat depression, but now considered disreputable. Amphetamines, or 'speed', cause a monoamine, called noradrenaline, which is stored in nerve endings to be released. The effect is to elevate the mood, abolish sleepiness, to appear to increase the capacity for work, and generally speed up mental action. The drug does not, however, improve performance of any kind and can be dangerous. It is used to a limited extent for a few special medical purposes but is subject to the full restrictions on controlled drugs laid down in the Misuse of Drugs Act (1971).

Anabolic steroids

These are drugs that cause an increase in body bulk by stimulating the production of protein, mainly in the muscles, but also elsewhere. They actually work inside cells, causing an acceleration of the processes by which amino acids in the cell fluid are strung together to form protein. Anabolic steroids are synthetic male sex hormone steroids such as ethyloestrenol, nandrolone, norethan-drolone and stanolone.

Their use may sometimes be justified to help elderly and under-weight people to gain strength and they can be valuable in women with the condition of seriously weakened bones known as osteo-porosis.

Some of the anabolic steroids, being male sex hormones, cause development of male characteristics in women. This is called viril-ization and may feature hairiness, wasting (atrophy) of the breasts, enlargement of the clitoris, deepening of the voice and severe acne. Anabolic steroids are widely used by body-building enthusiasts and athletes to improve muscle bulk and strength. This usage has right-ly been banned by sporting authorities, not only because of its unfairness to other competitors, but also because of the possible adverse effects on health. Among these are:

- virilization in women (see above)
- virilization of a female fetus
- increased libido
- frequent erections
- failure of an erection to go down (priapism)
- liver damage
- a dangerous and sometimes fatal form of heart enlargement
- major depression
- hallucinations
- religious delusions and delusions of grandeur
- aggressive or manic behaviour

Anabolic steroids can encourage the growth of an existing cancer of the prostate gland in men.

Anaesthetic drugs

Modern general anaesthetic drugs are designed to keep you lightly and safely asleep, while, at the same time, causing your muscles to relax completely so as not to interfere with the surgery. They are also selected to abolish pain sensation and produce a calm, relaxed state of mind, before and after the anaesthetic. Narcotic drugs, such as morphine, Omnopon or Valium (diazepam), are used before an operation (pre-medication), to promote your confidence, relax your muscles, help you to forget the unpleasantness, and keep you comfortable afterwards. These drugs act directly on the brain, safely and temporarily interfering with the function of the nerve cells that allow sensation, consciousness and movement. The drug atropine is often given to reduce the tendency for fluid to collect in your air tubes.

So, if you are having an operation, you are likely to be wheeled to theatre in a very comfortable frame of mind, if not already asleep. If you are awake when you reach the anaesthetic room, you are unlikely to be put to sleep with a mask and anaesthetic gas or vapour. Anaesthesia is almost always induced by a small injection into a vein of a rapid-acting drug, such as the barbiturate Pentothal (thiopentone). This is very pleasant and there is hardly any awareness of what is happening. Anaesthesia is maintained, at a very light level for safety, by means of inhaled drugs such as nitrous oxide or halothane. These are often combined with a strong pain-killing ANALGESIC DRUG because, although you are unconscious, stimuli which would otherwise be painful can still cause unwanted changes in your body.

Only after you are deeply asleep will the gases, which keep you anaesthetized, be turned on. There will be none of the sense of asphyxiation which was formerly a feature of general anaesthesia.

If muscle relaxation is needed, this is now achieved by one of a number of drugs which temporarily paralyze the muscles. In this event, your breathing must be maintained artificially. Sometimes blood pressure is deliberately lowered by ANTIHYPERTENSIVE DRUGS.

Analeptic drugs

These are drugs which stimulate the nerve centres in the brain responsible for breathing. Their action is to increase the strength of the nerve impulses going to the breathing muscles – the diaphragm and the muscles between the ribs (intercostal muscles). Analeptics, such as doxapram (Dopram) or nikethamide are used to stimulate poor or absent breathing in newborn babies and are sometimes used in cases of drug overdose when the victim is barely breathing, or to speed recovery from a general anaesthetic. The drug naloxone (Narcan), which is an antidote to narcotic drugs, while not an analeptic, is also commonly used in such cases.

Side effects of analeptic drugs include nausea and vomiting, restlessness, dizziness, fast pulse, irregular pulse, shakiness, tremor and even convulsions. They are dangerous in people with coronary artery disease, severe high blood pressure and thyroid gland over-activity.

Analgesic drugs

This is the important group of painkilling drugs. It includes a wide range of drugs from the mild and comparatively safe (in correct dosage), such as paracetamol (Panadol), to the powerful and dangerous, such as the narcotics.

Paracetamol

Paracetamol works mainly by blocking the passage of the nerve impulses for pain so that they do not reach the part of the brain where pain is perceived. In general, it is a safe painkiller, but paracetamol is a serious liver poison if many tablets are taken at once. Twenty tablets can cause severe liver damage. The victim seems fine for a few days, then begins to turn yellow from the jaundice of an often fatal total liver failure. Antidotes, if given early enough, are methionine or N-acetylcysteine (Parvolex).

NSAIDs

Most of the other mild analgesics, such as the non-steroidal anti-inflammatory drugs (NSAIDs), work in a different way. When tissue cells are injured in any way they release powerful substances called prostaglandins. Prostaglandins strongly stimulate pain nerve endings and the result is the experience of pain. NSAIDs act by blocking the production of prostaglandins. Some drugs, such as morphine, act directly on the brain; others, like paracetamol, act on nerve conduction. But the Aspirin-like drugs act directly on damaged cells and work solely by preventing the production of the substances which cause the pain. Aspirin has no effect on the pain of a needle-prick because this directly stimulates the pain nerve endings, nor has it any effect on the pain caused by an injection of prostaglandins.

The non-steroidal anti-inflammatory drugs include Aspirin, aloxiprin (Palaprin forte), benorylate (Benoral), diflunisal (Dolobid), mefenamic acid (Ponstan), fenbufen (Lederfen), fenoprofen (Progesic), ibuprofen (Brufen), naproxen (Naprosyn), diclofenac (Voltarol), tolmetin (Tolectin), indomethacin (Indocid), phenylbutazone (Butazolidin) and piroxicam (Feldene).

NSAIDs often cause side effects. About half of those taking them get some degree of tummy upset, with nausea and diarrhoea. They may also cause headache, sleep disturbances, allergic rashes and dizziness. Occasionally there can be interference with white blood cell (immune system cell) production. See also side effects of Aspirin.

Aspirin

Aspirin can cause quite severe irritation to the lining of the stomach. If you keep a tablet of plain Aspirin between your cheek and your gum for half an hour, it will turn the mucous membrane white and wrinkled and will loosen the surface. Aspirin can do the same to your stomach lining, causing congestion and bleeding around undissolved particles. Over half of all people taking Aspirin have traces of blood in their faeces. So you should never use plain Aspirin. Only the soluble variety, which rapidly breaks up and dissolves, is safe. If you suffer from indigestion or have a previous history of ulcer trouble you should avoid Aspirin altogether.

Following a virus infection in children, Aspirin can cause a serious liver and brain disorder called Reye's syndrome. So Aspirin is no longer given to children. Aspirin allergy is rare but may occur in people with other allergies. It can cause alarming and often dangerous reactions, including severe breathing difficulty. Aspirin and the NSAIDs interfere with blood clotting and prolong bleeding. This can be very useful in preventing heart attacks (which are caused by blood clotting in the coronary arteries of the heart). But it can sometimes be dangerous. People with a tendency to stroke might be saved from a cerebral thrombosis (clot), but might be at greater risk from a more serious cerebral haemorrhage. A minor eye injury with a small leak of blood into the front chamber can be turned into an eye-filling bleed by a single Aspirin tablet, which doubles the bleeding time for up to a week.

Intermediate analgesics
An intermediate group of analgesics consists of a mixture of these mild analgesics with the mild – and fairly safe – narcotic analgesic, codeine. There is a large range of proprietary medications consisting of various combinations of codeine, Aspirin and various NSAIDs. Other moderately potent narcotic drugs, unlikely to cause addiction, are dihydrocodeine, pentazocine and dextropropoxyphene.

Narcotic analgesics
For the relief of very severe pain, more powerful narcotic drugs may be needed. These are used only when other drugs are ineffective, and include morphine, phenazocine and methadone. The narcotic analgesics act on specific receptor sites, called opiate receptors, in the brain and spinal cord, blocking the pain sensation. The natural endorphins of the body act in the same way. These strong narcotic analgesics also produce a powerful feeling of wellbeing (euphoria) and are abused for this reason. They are strongly addictive. Heroin (diamorphine), formerly widely used in medicine, is now banned in most countries because of this danger.

Angina

Angina pectoris, to give it its full name, is not a disease but a symptom. It is the strong burning and constricting sensation felt in the chest when the heart muscle needs more oxygen than its blood supply can provide. This usually occurs when your heart is required to speed up to perform work, such as occurs when you walk a certain distance or climbing stairs. Strong emotion, too, can speed up the heart and cause angina. Sometimes, in severe cases, angina may occur even at rest, but usually some exertion is needed. Often the degree is well known to the sufferer.

Your heart muscle gets its blood supply through the coronary arteries, which are branches of the large artery coming directly out of the top of the heart. If the coronary arteries are severely narrowed by disease – usually atherosclerosis – they may not be able to pass enough blood to meet the needs of the rapidly beating heart. Most of the blood flow through the coronaries occurs between the heart beats, when the arteries are not compressed by the contracting muscle. The result of a faster heart rate, therefore, is to allow less time for the blood to flow. This is one reason why angina is always more likely when the heart beats fast and why it is rare in heart disease that causes a slow pulse. Sometimes angina is caused by tight contraction of the tiny circular muscles in the walls of the coronary arteries. This is called coronary spasm and severely restricts the blood flow.

The speed of your heart, and the force of the contractions are controlled by nerves from the sympathetic nervous system and by the hormone adrenaline. These, in turn, are activated by the demands made by your body and the mind. One important group of drugs for angina make the heart less sensitive to stimuli from the sympathetic system and from adrenaline. These are the beta-adrenergic blocking agents, commonly known as the BETA BLOCKER DRUGS. They slow the heart rate and reduce the force of the contraction, so the need for oxygen is less. The beta blockers are very valuable, but they are for long-term use and it is dangerous suddenly to stop taking them. If they bring your heart rate, while you are resting, down below about 55 beats per minute, you may be having too high a dose. Tell your doctor.

In an emergency, the supply of blood through your coronary arteries can be temporarily increased by widening them. A drug which does this very effectively is nitroglycerin (glyceryl trinitrate). This is absorbed from a tablet placed under the tongue. There are longer-acting nitrates, such as isosorbide dinitrate, and these may be used to try to prevent angina (see ARTERY-WIDENING DRUGS). Another new and very useful group of drugs are the CALCIUM CHANNEL BLOCKER DRUGS. These reduce the force of the heart beat, widen the coronary arteries and reduce the load on the heart by also widening other arteries in the body so that the general resistance to blood flow is reduced. They are especially valuable if there is suspicion that angina is being caused by spasm of the coronary arteries.

Angiotensin converting enzyme inhibitors

The name of this group is a real mouthful, so they are usually known as the ACE inhibitors. The kidneys produce a chemical activator (enzyme) called renin. This cuts off a piece of protein called angiotensin I from a larger blood protein. Angiotensin I doesn't do very much, but there is another enzyme in the blood called the angiotensin converting enzyme (ACE), and this converts angiotensin I to the powerfully active angiotensin II. Angiotensin II causes arteries to narrow and this raises the blood pressure. An inhibitor is something that stops something else from acting. So ACE inhibitors prevent ACE from turning the harmless angiotensin I into the active angiotensin II. They thus lower blood pressure and improve blood flow. These drugs are valuable in the management of high blood pressure (hypertension) and certain forms of heart failure.

ACE inhibitors include captopril (Acepril, Acezide, Capoten, Capozide) and enalapril (Vasotec, Innovace, Innozide). About 10% of people taking these drugs get skin rashes and some suffer disturbances of taste sensation. Minor kidney damage can occur. About one person in 300 suffers interference with white blood cell production. In rare cases this may be very severe.

Antacid drugs

These are drugs that reduce or neutralize excess acid in your stomach and relieve the symptoms of heartburn. Heartburn is the result of acid being pushed up from the stomach into the gullet. This is called acid reflux.

Stomach and duodenal ulcers (open sores in the inner lining) are grouped together as peptic ulcers. These are caused by the action of stomach acid and the digestive protein-splitting enzyme, pepsin, on the inner lining. Pepsin only works in the presence of acid. Your stomach lining is normally protected by a layer of mucus, produced by many cells in the lining. Any defect in this mucous layer allows the pepsin to start digesting the wall. Smoking and the over-use of irritating drugs like strong alcohol, Aspirin and Brufen are among the causes of a defect in the protective mucus layer. The more acid present the more likely are you to start digesting yourself.

The part of the bowel immediately beyond your stomach is called the duodenum. This contains alkaline secretions which can neutralize normal quantities of stomach acid. So duodenal ulcers only occur if there is excess of acid and pepsin. If the acid levels can be kept low enough neither stomach nor duodenal ulcers will occur. This can be done in two ways – by preventing the acid from being produced by the use of drugs such as cimetidine or ranitidine, or by chemically neutralising the acid once it has been produced. The drugs which do the latter are called antacids.

The most popular and cheapest antacid is the alkali baking soda (sodium bicarbonate). This acts quickly and gives you rapid relief of pain. Unfortunately, the acid acts on the bicarbonate to produce volumes of carbon dioxide gas, and much belching results. The bicarbonate is also absorbed into your blood and too much of it can make your blood alkaline – which can be serious. Other antacids include magnesium oxide, magnesium hydroxide and magnesium trisilicate. These are not absorbed, but the first two act as purgatives. Magnesium trisilicate works more slowly than the oxides and you need quite large doses, but in addition to neutralizing the acid, it also inactivates the pepsin and is fairly effective. Aluminium hydroxide (Aludrox) also binds the pepsin and neutralises the acid. It, too, must be taken in large dosage for full effect. Antacids may also provide a protective coating to the lining of the stomach and duodenum.

Like the rest of the stomach contents, antacids are quickly passed out of the stomach. About half has gone in half an hour. So it is not really satisfactory to take them only when pain is felt – as most people do. Of course, the management of dyspepsia and peptic ulcers involves more than just the use of antacids. Self-treatment is not always safe.

H_2 receptor antagonists

Histamine is a powerful and important hormone found in most of your body tissues in inactivated form, mainly in cells called mast cells. Histamine is released when cells are injured, either physically or as a result of an allergic reaction. It affects other cells by way of cell *receptors* and has various actions. It causes the muscle in the walls of the air tubes of the lungs to tighten, it causes arteries to widen, small blood vessels (capillaries) to leak, skin to itch and the lining of the stomach to secrete acid. There are two kinds of histamine receptors – H_1 and H_2. H_1 receptor antagonists block the effects of histamine produced as a result of allergic or other reactions and are called ANTIHISTAMINE DRUGS. The H_2 receptor antagonists operate mainly in the stomach lining and to a lesser extent in the walls of the arteries.

A group of drugs known as the H_2 receptor antagonists has revolutionized the treatment of stomach and duodenal ulcers. These drugs act by blocking action of histamine on the H_2 receptors and thus cutting down the secretion of acid. This important class of drugs includes cimetidine (Tagamet, Algitec, Dyspamet, Galenamet) and ranitidine (Zantac). These drugs have made a fortune for the manufacturers. They are so effective that doctors have to be very careful to ensure a correct diagnosis before using them as they can actually, for a time, relieve the symptoms of cancer of the stomach. They do not, of course, have any effect on the growth of cancer, and what may seem like successful treatment may lead to dangerous delay.

The H_2 receptor antagonists are also valuable in the management of heartburn, stress ulcers in people with severe burns and the Zollinger-Ellison syndrome. This is a condition caused by a hormone-secreting tumour of the pancreas, known as a gastrinoma. This tumour produces large quantities of the hormone gastrin, which powerfully stimulates acid production in the stomach. The result is a massive outpouring of stomach acid, inevitably leading to severe ulceration of the stomach and duodenum (peptic ulceration).

The H_2 receptor antagonists have few side effects, apart from the possible concealment of stomach cancer, and these are minor. They include diarrhoea or constipation, tiredness, headache, muscle pain, and slowing of the heart. Cimetidine is mildly antagonistic to the male sex hormones and may cause enlargement of the breasts in men and, possibly, impotence. Ranitidine does not have this effect.

There is one additional important thing to be said about peptic ulceration. There is increasing evidence that the organism *Helicobacter pylori*, which is found in the bowels of a high proportion of people suffering from peptic ulceration, has a significant role to play in the causation of duodenal ulcer. Destruction of this organism with bismuth in association with amoxycillin and metronidazole is usually followed by healing of ulcers. Bismuth causes these organisms to detach from the bowel lining. The use of these drugs, especially bismuth, appears to be capable of preventing recurrence. Ask your doctor about this. Bismuth can turn the inside of your mouth black, and, like iron, can also cause black faeces. Don't forget, however, that this can be caused by bleeding from the stomach.

The H₂ receptor antagonists have few side effects. Ranitidine is especially free from adverse effects. See also PROTON PUMP INHIBITOR DRUGS.

Antagonist drug

Any drug that opposes the action of another drug or of a natural body substance such as a hormone.

Anthelmintic drugs

These are drugs used to rid the body of parasitic worms. Different kinds of drugs are used to kill or paralyse different worms and it is important to identify the type of worm before starting treatment. Paralysed worms let go of the lining of the bowel, or the tissues, and either pass out with the faeces or may, if necessary, be removed surgically from tissues. Sometimes a laxative is given with the anthelmintic drug to help evacuate intestinal worms.

Commonly used anthelmintic drugs include piperazine (Pripsen) for roundworms and threadworms; tetrachloroethylene or thiabendazole (Mintezol) for hookworms; niclosamide or praziquantel for tapeworms; niridazole or metronidazole (Flagyl) for guinea worm; diethylcarbamazine for filariasis; praziquantel for schistosomiasis; mebendazole (Vermox) for whipworm; and diethylcarbamazine (Banocide) or thiabendazole (Mintezol) for toxocariasis (larva migrans).

Most anthelmintic drugs can cause abdominal discomfort, nausea and vomiting. Metronidazole is remarkably free from side effects, but long-term treatment can sometimes cause nerve problems. It reacts badly with alcohol to cause severe symptoms similar to those caused by Antabuse.

Antiamoebic drugs

Drugs able to destroy or suppress amoebae of medical importance, especially the amoeba that causes amoebic dysentery, include emetine, metronidazole (Flagyl), tinidazole (Fasigyn) and chloroquine (Aclochlor, Nivaquine).

Antiandrogen drugs

This is a group of drugs given in rare circumstances to sexually criminal men to dampen down their urges by interfering with the action of their male sex hormones. Antiandrogen dugs are also used in cases of cancer of the prostate gland. The group include cyproterone acetate (Androcur, Cyprostat), cimetidine (Tagamet) and spironolactone. Antiandrogen drugs may cause breast enlargement (gynaecomastia).

Antianxiety drugs

You can't really separate severe anxiety from the physical effects that are associated with it – muscle tension, tremor, sweating and a fast heart rate. Some scientists even believe that these symptoms are actually the *cause* of the anxiety, rather than the effect. Certainly, any drug which controls these symptoms will relieve the level of anxiety and may even temporarily abolish it. Antianxiety drugs, often rather fancifully called 'anxiolytics' are, in general, minor sedatives and tranquillizers that relax muscles and slow the heart. They include beta-blockers, such as propranolol (Inderal, Betadur) and oxprenolol, and BENZODIAZEPINE DRUGS, such as diazepam (Valium) and chlordiazepoxide (Librium). BARBITURATES are seldom used nowadays.

Antianxiety drugs, although useful, are not, of course, the definitive treatment for anxiety. For this, you need help to study the life problems and reactions underlying the anxiety and the benefit of the skilled counselling and advice of a wise psychotherapist. Some forms of anxiety, especially those associated with phobias, are probably best treated by behaviour therapy.

Like any other sedatives, the antianxiety drugs are liable to increase the effects of alcohol.

Antiarrhythmia drugs

These are drugs used to control irregularities of the heartbeat. They include digitalis and quinidine, which have been in use for many decades, procainamide, BETA-BLOCKER DRUGS, CALCIUM CHANNEL BLOCKER DRUGS and disopyramide. These drugs act in different ways to convert irregular and inefficient contractions into steady, slower and more forceful beats, thereby improving the pumping efficiency of the heart.

Antibiotic drugs

This is one of the largest groups of drugs and one of the best known. It is impossible to compute the benefits conferred on humanity by the antibiotics. Sixty years ago, medicine was dominated by bacterial infection, which was the major cause of death and was responsible for an immense amount of suffering, long-term ill-health and disability. Parents would listen with alarm to their children's coughing or contemplate with terror red streaks running up the arm from a septic area. Enlarged lymph nodes ('glands') could be a prelude to blood poisoning (septicaemia). Compound fractures of limbs often led to amputation. A squeezed pustule on the nose might cause a spreading fatal infection into the brain. Lobar pneumonia was commonplace and often fatal, and osteomyelitis (bone marrow infection) caused discharging channels (sinuses) for years. Tuberculosis sanitoria were full of people coughing up blood and sputum.

All that has changed and most people alive today have no concept of a world without antibiotics. These drugs kill germs (microorganisms) in the body, or prevent their growth or reproduction. As a result, almost all diseases caused by infecting bacteria can now be cured by antibiotics. You should appreciate, however, that antibiotics have *no* effect on viruses. Antibiotics were originally derived from cultures of living organisms, such as fungi or bacteria, but, today, many can be chemically synthesized.

There are many antibiotics and the multiplication of official and trade names is bewildering, but they fall into groups, and the members of each group are related chemically, or by derivation, to each other. These groups are:

- the penicillins (penicillin G, penicillin V, cloxacillin, flucloxacillin and many others)
- the cephalosporins (cephaloridin, cephalothin, cefuroxime and many others)
- the aminoglycosides (gentamicin, streptomycin, tobramycin, netilmicin, amikacin, neomycin and framycetin)
- the tetracyclines (tetracycline, chlortetracycline – aureomycin, methacycline, oxytetracycline – terramycin and others)
- the imidazoles (metronidazole – flagyl, ketoconazole, miconazole, nimorazole, mebendazole and thiabendazole)

In addition to these, there are other individual antibiotics such as chloramphenicol, erythromycin, lincomycin, clindamycin and spectinomycin.

Bacteriologists and others commonly criticize the way some doctors use antibiotics. There is some justification for the view that occasionally doctors prescribe them needlessly or for trivial infections. Sometimes, this misuse stems from pressure from patients who demand antibiotics. Sometimes it occurs because busy doctors feel they can't take chances with infections that might become serious, but which they do not have time to investigate as thoroughly as they might. Some hospital doctors, more concerned with the immediate pressing needs of their patients than with the possible future hazards to society as a whole, do sometimes prescribe powerful new drugs when safer, established, remedies would suffice. The two essential problems are the development of strains of bacteria resistant to antibiotics and the risk of undesirable side effects.

If antibiotics are used casually and in inadequate dosage – and this is not always the doctor's fault – the bacteria which are most sensitive to the drug will be killed while those which happen to have a natural genetic resistance will survive. When the latter reproduce, new strains of resistant organisms result. This process of natural selection is accelerated by the brevity of the bacterial generation – only about 20 minutes in ideal conditions. As a result of this process many organisms are now resistant to antibiotics that formerly were effective against them. This has put heavy pressures on research workers to produce new antibiotics and keep ahead. So today, we have an on-going race between the development of resistance in bacteria, on the one hand, and the development of new antibiotics, on the other. We should be grateful to the men and women of the pharmaceutical industry who, so far, have enabled us to keep ahead in the race. You will now appreciate that, ideally, antibiotics should be used only for serious, or potentially serious infections or to prevent dangerous conditions in specially susceptible people. If you are prescribed a course of antibiotics, you should take it completely and regularly.

Powerful antibiotics often produce undesirable side effects. These include:

- allergies, especially to penicillin, which may be serious or even fatal
- deafness, permanent ringing or hissing in the ears (tinnitus), kidney damage or interference with normal blood production (aminoglycoside antibiotics)
- permanent staining of teeth (tetracycline antibiotics, if given to young children)
- destruction of normal, health-giving body bacteria
- over-growth of undesirable organisms such as the candida fungus that causes thrush
- nausea, intestinal upset and diarrhoea
- skin rashes

It would be naive to suppose that infections have been conquered. Many people still die from infections, and none of these side effects will deter doctors from giving what is often life-saving therapy.

Anticancer drugs

Most anticancer drugs are cytotoxic drugs – that is, drugs that destroy rapidly growing cells, but some are sex hormones or similar substances. Cytotoxic drugs are especially useful in the treatment of some forms of leukaemia, lymphomas, and cancers of the testicle and ovary. They are often used as an additional safeguard after surgery or in conjunction with radiotherapy. Cytotoxic drugs cause more damage to cancer cells than normal body cells. In most cases the drug can distinguish cancer cells from other cells by the speed with which cancer cells reproduce. Normal cells are restrained in their ability to multiply; cancer cells have lost some or all of this restraint. Cytotoxic drugs are most active against cells which are not restrained in this way. Unfortunately, the ability to distinguish between the two types is not complete and cytotoxic drugs cannot avoid causing some damage to normal cells. Consequently they always have major side effects.

The more rapidly normal cells reproduce, the more likely they are to be damaged by cytotoxic drugs. For this reason, these drugs cause most damage to cells in the lining of the bowel, hair-producing cells, the sex glands and the blood forming tissue in the bone marrow. The typical side effects thus include:

- nausea and vomiting
- hair loss
- sterility
- anaemia and a tendency to bleeding

People treated with these drugs always have a frequent check made of their red and white blood cell counts. Cytotoxic drugs include chlorambucil (Leukeran), cyclophosphamide (Endoxana), lomustine (CCNU), methotrexate (Maxtrex), vinblastine, vincristine, adriamycin, bleomycin and nitrogen mustard. However you look at it, these are unpleasant substances and people taking them have a bad time. But doctors would not use them if there were better ways of attacking the cancer.

Some cancers are 'hormone dependent'. This means that certain hormones make them grow faster. Thus, some kinds of breast cancer are stimulated to grow by the female sex hormones known as oestrogens. This means that they can be discouraged from growing by male sex hormones – which oppose oestrogens – or by the drug tamoxifen which also has anti-oestrogenic properties. Paradoxically, the growth of some breast cancers, especially in elderly women, is *discouraged* by oestrogen hormones given in very high doses. In men, the common cancer of the prostate gland is male hormone dependent and can often be greatly diminished by treatment with a female sex hormone such as stilboestrol.

Anticholinergic drugs

The autonomic nervous system is the collection of nerves concerned with the non-voluntary control of many body functions. The autonomic system has two generally opposing parts – the sympathetic, concerned with emergency situations (fright, fight and flight) and the parasympathetic, concerned with calm situations. Adrenaline is the sympathetic hormone and acetylcholine is the parasympathetic hormone. Acetylcholine is released at many nerve endings in the parasympathetic and has many effects. These include constriction of the pupils, contraction of the bladder wall, relaxation of controlling muscle rings (sphincters), the production of saliva, tears, sweat and respiratory secretions, slowing of the heart, narrowing of the air tubes and increasing the activity of the bowels. These acetylcholine effects are called 'cholinergic'. Anticholinergic drugs are drugs that block the receptors for acetylcholine. They have, of course, a considerable range of effects which you can work out for yourself. They cause a dry mouth, dry eyes, a dry, hot skin, widely-dilated pupils, a rapid heartbeat, relief of bowel colic and difficulty in emptying the bladder. The classic anticholinergic drug is belladonna (atropine).

Such atropine-like drugs are useful in drying up secretions prior to an operation, treating an unduly slow heart rate, and relieving the symptoms of the irritable bowel syndrome and certain types of urinary incontinence. They are also used to treat Parkinson's disease, asthma, and MOTION SICKNESS. Overdosage, in addition to the effects mentioned, also causes:

- difficulty in swallowing
- retention of urine

- blurred vision
- anxiety
- delirium
- hallucinations
- confusion and convulsions

Apart from atropine itself, other anticholinergic drugs are hyoscine (Buscopan), scopolamine (the same as hyoscine), homatropine, banthine, propantheline (Pro-Banthine) and dibutoline.

Anticoagulant drugs

Blood clotting is essential to prevent continuous loss of blood from wounds. But blood clotting *within* the blood vessels is very dangerous and is one of the main causes of death. Anticoagulant drugs reduce the normal tendency of blood to clot and can prevent clots forming in the circulation (thromboses). They can also prevent existing clots from getting bigger. They do not reduce the size of clots which have already formed. Anticoagulants work better in the veins than in the arteries and are most useful in the prevention and treatment of deep vein thrombosis. They are important in the prevention of clot formation on artificial heart valves or when an artificial kidney (dialysis machine) is in use. One of the most valuable uses of anticoagulant drugs is to prevent long, soft, snakelike clots forming in the deep leg veins of people immobilized after surgery or for other reasons. These loose clots are very dangerous as they can break off and be carried up through the heart to the lungs where they clog the main arteries carrying blood to the lungs. This is called pulmonary embolism and it is a common cause of death.

The most important anticoagulant drug is the body's own natural anticoagulant, heparin. This is still the most generally useful drug and is sold as Clexane, Fragmin, Hepsal, Minihep, Monoparin, etc. Heparin blocks the activity of various coagulation factors needed for the clotting of the blood. It must be given by injection at least every six hours and it begins to work within a few hours. Other anticoagulant drugs may be taken by mouth but are slow to take effect. Often these are started along with heparin, and the heparin injections stopped after three days. Oral anticoagulants include warfarin, nicoumalone, phenindione and the antiplatelet drugs protamine sulphate, dipyridamole and sulphinpyrazone.

Anticoagulant drugs must be used with great care and with constant monitoring of the blood-clotting tendency to avoid the risk of severe internal bleeding. Nevertheless, they have saved many lives.

Anticonvulsant drugs

These drugs are used to prevent epileptic seizures and must be taken continuously for long periods, usually twice a day. A single drug, rather than a combination, is usually preferred and the dose given is the least which achieves the objective. A second drug may have to be added if one fails to prevent attacks.

Anticonvulsant drugs are used in cases of established epilepsy, in certain cases of head injury in which there is a tendency to seizures, in the emergency treatment of a prolonged seizure and sometimes to prevent seizures in children with a history of fits during fevers (febrile seizures).

The choice of drug depends on the type of seizure and on the person's response. Most cases of epilepsy can be well controlled with one or other of the commonly used drugs. Phenobarbitone (Luminal), phenytoin (Dilantin), carbamazepine (Tegretol), and primidone (Mysoline) will control major fits ('grand mal') and the local twitching known as focal epilepsy. Phenobarbitone, ethosuximide (Zarontin), and methsuximide (Celontin) are effective in the repeated childhood 'switching-off' known as 'petit mal' or absence attacks. Valproic acid (Depakene) and clonazepam (Rivotril) are valuable in absence and partial seizures.

The doctor must carefully adjust the dosage to give the least necessary to prevent attacks. Sometimes a combination of two drugs gives better results than one alone. Overdosage, which can cause mental dullness, even stupefaction, must, of course, be avoided. When major attacks occur one after the other, diazepam (Valium) is given by injection until the seizures stop. This dangerous but fortunately rare complication is called status epilepticus.

Antidepressant drugs

The treatment of depression involves more than just prescribing drugs, but effective treatments do exist and most affected people can be greatly helped, however severe their depression.

One of the basic facts about the nervous system is that messages (nerve impulses) are passed on from one nerve to another by means of a tiny quantity of a powerful chemical substance called a neuro-transmitter. This substance floats across the gap between the two nerves and causes the second nerve to send on an impulse. There are many different neurotransmitters in the body, but among the most important are substances, similar to adrenaline, called monoamines. Depression is often caused by a shortage, or decreased effectiveness, of monoamines at the nerve endings. Too much monoamine and you get overactivity – causing elation, an exaggerated sense of wellbeing, even mania. Not enough, and you get black depression.

The drug amphetamine, or 'speed', causes a monoamine called noradrenaline, which is stored in nerve endings, to be released. Everyone knows the effect. In fact, amphetamine was once widely used to treat depression, until its undesirable side effects, and the probability of its being abused, became widely known.

Monoamine oxidase inhibitors (MAOI)

Do not be put off by this complicated name. The explanation is quite simple. Monoamines in the nerve endings are kept under control by a breaking-down chemical (enzyme) called monoamine oxidase. Drugs that interfere with the action of this enzyme are called monoamine oxidase inhibitors. These drugs are packaged for the treatment of depression under such names as Marplan, Marsilid, Nardil and Parnate. They are quite useful when depression is accompanied by much anxiety and phobias, but they, too, have some disadvantages and are not usually given as the first line of treatment. For instance, they interfere with the breakdown of the common monoamine (amino acid) tyramine that is found in cheese, chocolate, alcohol, yeast extracts such as Marmite, meat extracts and other foods. If you are taking monoamine oxidase inhibitors you must not eat any of these foods, because the result will be an abnormally high level of tyramine. This can dangerously raise your blood pressure.

Tricyclic antidepressants
When the monoamine neurotransmitters have triggered a new nerve impulse, they are not destroyed but drift away from the receptor sites and are then pumped back into their original nerve endings. This pumping action can be chemically blocked, so that more monoamine remains around – exactly what we need. The substances that do this are called tricyclic antidepressants, and this group contains the most valuable drugs for depression. They are marketed under names such as Anafranil, Aventyl, Domical, Evadyne, Lentizol, Saroten, Sinequan, Tofranil and Tryptizol. There are dozens more. It is essential for you to appreciate that all the tricyclics take from ten to fourteen days, sometimes longer, to have a worthwhile action. After that time, however, their effect may seem miraculous. They do have side effects, however, that you should know about. The tricyclics can cause:

- dryness of the mouth
- difficulty with urination
- delayed ejaculation in men
- angle-closure glaucoma in susceptible people
- difficulty in focusing the eyes

They can also sometimes interfere with the action of the heart, can make epilepsy worse, and can interfere with the control of diabetes. Different members of the group have these effects to different degrees, so the doctor must choose carefully which to prescribe.

Antidiabetic drugs
There are two kind of diabetes. Type I usually starts in childhood or adolescence and is due to destruction of the insulin-producing cells in the pancreas. Type II comes on later and is due to insufficient insulin production relative to needs. People with Type I diabetes are

known as 'insulin-dependent' diabetics; those with Type II diabetes are 'non-insulin dependent', or 'maturity-onset' diabetics. Much of the food we eat is converted to the body fuel glucose (sugar). Diabetics cannot properly use this glucose and it accumulates in the blood and appears in the urine. Insulin allows muscle and other cells to use glucose normally. Too little insulin and the blood sugar level rises; too much, and it falls dangerously. The amount of insulin needed by insulin-dependent diabetics depends on the amount of food taken and the rate it is used up by exertion. The only way to be sure that the right amount of insulin is being taken is to check the blood sugar levels directly by means of a small machine.

Insulin used to be obtained from pigs and oxen, and much animal insulin is still used. But genetic engineering has now made it easy to produce genuine human insulin without involving animals at all. Human insulins, such as Humulin, are being increasingly used. Insulin has to be taken by injection and there are many preparations. Some have a quick and immediate effect, some have a more prolonged effect. Mixtures of different preparations of insulins are often used. There is a great deal more to the subject than this, and if you are a diabetic you will certainly know a great deal more than I can cover here. Diabetics cannot know too much about the condition.

Type II diabetes can often be controlled on diet alone, especially if the insulin supply is inadequate only because you are overweight. Often, however, it is necessary to go further and to take drugs of the group known as the oral hypoglycaemics. This just means that you take them by mouth and they reduce your blood sugar levels. There are two kinds of oral hypoglycaemics – the sulphonylureas and the biguanides. The sulphonureas, which include tolbutamide, chlor-propamide and glibenclamide, act by stimulating the pancreas to produce more insulin. The biguanides are drugs such as metformin and phenformin. They work by interfering with the absorption of carbohydrates from the intestine, by reducing the production of glucose by the liver and by increasing the utilization of glucose fuel by the tissues. None of the oral hypoglycaemic drugs are any good if the pancreas is not producing any insulin. In such a case, the person concerned must have insulin injections.

Antidiarrhoeal drugs

Diarrhoea nearly always serves the useful purpose of flushing out irritants from the bowel, such as infecting germs. So it is not a good idea to take a drug to check it as soon as it starts. In most cases, nature will solve the problem unaided, but if diarrhoea persists for more than two or three days, it usually needs to be treated.

Drugs to check diarrhoea may either be narcotics like codeine, which reduce the irritability of the bowel wall and cut down the rate of contraction of the bowel muscles, or substances, such as methyl cellulose or a high fibre diet, which increase the bulk and solidity of the bowel contents. Other substances, such as chalk, ispaghula husk or kaolin, can be useful. Narcotic preparations include codeine, diphenoxylate (Lomotil), loperamide (Imodium), kaolin and morphine mixture, and aromatic chalk and opium.

Antidote

An antidote is a drug that neutralizes or counteracts the action or effect of a poison. There are few specific antidotes. These include naloxone for narcotic opiate poisoning, desferrioxamine for iron poisoning, cobalt edetate for cyanide poisoning, and methionine and n-acetylcysteine for paracetamol poisoning. Activated charcoal may be valuable to adsorb poisons.

All this means that for most cases of poisoning there are *no* antidotes, and valuable time can be wasted trying to find out about them. Turn to Chapter 6 for guidance on the subject of poisoning and for the telephone numbers of poisons centres in the UK and Republic of Ireland.

Antiemetic drugs

Severe and prolonged nausea is very unpleasant. When combined with persistent vomiting it can be intolerable. Antiemetic drugs are drugs used to relieve nausea and prevent vomiting from any cause. They are useful in the control of motion sickness, for nausea associated with various kinds of vertigo including the symptoms of Ménière's disease, and the nausea associated with medical treatment with ANTICANCER DRUGS and other toxic drugs or sometimes with radiotherapy. They are valuable in the management of the nausea and vomiting of kidney failure (uraemia), widespread cancer, radiation sickness, and acute gastro-enteritis caused by viruses. Antiemetic drugs can often be given by mouth, but if the vomiting is severe, they will have to be given by injection or by a rectal suppository.

It is not good medicine to use antiemetic drugs to treat nausea and vomiting caused by a disease, when there is an effective remedy for the cause. The right thing to do in such a case is to treat the cause. Antiemetic drugs are also best avoided when the cause of the vomiting is unknown as their use may conceal the cause and preclude proper treatment. They are seldom used in diseases of the intestines, for instance.

ANTIHISTAMINE DRUGS, such as cyclizine, and ANTICHOLINERGIC DRUGS, such as hyoscine, can act as antiemetics by dampening down nerve impulses from the balancing mechanisms in the inner ears. Other antiemetics include atropine, chlorpromazine (Largactil), prochlorperazine (Stemetil), perphenazine (Fentazin), trifluoperazine (Stelazine), and ondansetron (Zofran).

Antifibrinolysis

Blood clotting, which prevents bleeding, can be very important. Clots are formed mainly from a network of strands of a material called fibrin. This can sometimes be broken down so that the clot ceases to seal off a wound. Such breaking down of a clot is called fibrinolysis. Drugs that prevent the breakdown of fibrin are called antifibrinolytic drugs. The most important of these are aminocaproic acid and tranexamic acid (Cyklokapron).

These drugs are used to control undue bleeding after surgery such as prostatectomy or to prevent prolonged bleeding after dental extraction in haemophiliacs. They can, however, cause complications such as blood clotting in the kidney urine drainage tubes with possible blockage. There is a risk of thrombosis if they are used in conjunction with oral contraceptives.

Antifungal drugs

These are drugs that act directly on the cell walls of the various fungi that infect the skin and, less commonly, the internal organs.

Antifungal drugs may be applied directly to the skin or mucous membranes in the form of creams, lotions, solutions or powders, or may be taken by mouth. For very severe internal fungal infections, antifungal drugs may have to be given by injection.

Antifungal drugs are used to treat the various kinds of tinea – athlete's foot (tinea pedis), body 'ringworm' (tinea corporis), scalp tinea (tinea capitis) and jock itch (tinea cruris); they are used to control thrush (candidiasis), whether of the skin, the vagina, the mouth or the internal organs; and they are used to try to control a number of rare internal fungus infections, such as cryptococcosis or torulopsosis.

Local applications include clotrimazole (Canesten), miconazole, econazole and nystatin (Nystan). Major antifungal drugs, for internal use, include amphotericin (Fungilin), flucytosine (Alcobon) and griseofulvin (Grisovin).

Given by injection, the imidazole antifungal drugs are apt to cause vein irritation and local thrombosis. This route may also be associated with nausea, vomiting, fever and rashes. By mouth they cause little trouble, but may occasionally lead to nausea, vomiting, diarrhoea, skin itching and sometimes hepatitis. They should be stopped at once if the skin turns yellow (jaundice).

Antihistamine drugs

Histamine is a powerful agent produced in the body by certain cells called *mast cells*, especially as an allergic response. It acts on small blood vessels, causing them to widen and allow the leakage of proteins so that these escape into the tissue fluid and cause swelling (oedema). The antihistamine group of drugs act against histamine and thus are useful in the treatment of many allergic conditions including hay fever (allergic rhinitis), asthma, urticaria, and other allergic rashes. They are commonly incorporated into cold and cough remedies because of their symptomatic effect and are valuable in the suppression of vomiting.

Side effects are common with antihistamine drugs and include:

- sedation
- sleepiness

- loss of coordination
- blurred vision
- dizziness
- loss of appetite
- nausea
- constipation
- dry mouth and difficulty in passing urine
- worsening of some kinds of glaucoma
- rarely, tremor, nervousness and insomnia

The list of antihistamines is long, but among the most important are diphenhydramine (Benadryl), promethazine (Phenergan), chlorpheniramine (Piriton), brompheniramine (Dimotane), clemastine (Tavegil), cyproheptadine (Periactin), dimethindene (Fenostil), diphenylpyraline (Histryl), mepyramine (Anthisan), phenindamine (Thephorin), and triprolidine (Actidil).

Antihypertensive drugs

These are drugs used for the control of abnormally raised blood pressure (hypertension). They are important because untreated hypertension can lead to complications such as stroke, heart attack, heart failure and kidney damage. Unfortunately, high blood pressure produces obvious symptoms only when it is severe or has already reached a fairly advanced stage and has caused damage to the blood vessels and the heart. So it has to be looked for. Every adult should have regular checks. Proper and effective treatment can largely eliminate the additional risk of these serious complications.

Three main classes of drugs are used to treat high blood pressure. The first, the DIURETIC DRUGS, act on the kidneys to cause them to pass more water and salt in the urine and reduce the volume of the blood, so bringing down the pressure. The second group, the BETA-BLOCKER DRUGS, interfere with the hormone and nervous control of the heart, slowing it and causing it to beat less forcefully, so reducing the pressure. The third group, the vasodilators, act on the arteries to widen them. This group contains drugs acting in quite different ways. They include the alpha blockers, the CALCIUM CHANNEL BLOCKER DRUGS and the ANGIOTENSIN-CONVERTING ENZYME INHIBITOR DRUGS.

The treatment of high blood pressure is not simply a matter of prescribing tablets. The doctor has difficult and complex decisions to make. Among others, he or she has to decide whether to use drugs at all. The body may have adapted to raised blood pressure, and reducing it may actually cause the person concerned to feel worse, rather than better. Until the body readjusts to normal pressures, there may be a sense of weakness and loss of energy, depression and a tendency to dizziness or faintness on standing up. The doctor aims to achieve control with the minimum dosage and will want to monitor the pressure regularly. Many other factors besides drugs are important in the treatment of high blood pressure. These include weight control, exercise and the avoidance of smoking.

Anti-inflammatory drugs

Inflammation is the commonest effect of injury to body tissues. It occurs as a result of a wide range of injurious processes including mechanical injury, burns, radiation, infection and poisons. It is essentially a reaction of small blood vessels which widen in response to injury, giving rise to the principal features of inflammation. These are:

- redness
- heat
- pain
- swelling
- loss of function

Inflammation is usually a protective reaction on the part of the body and it promotes effective action by the immune system and other bodily systems to combat the cause. It is not, therefore, always a good idea to combat inflammation. The correct order of procedure is to find the cause of the inflammation and, if possible, to eliminate it. There are, however, many circumstances in which inflammation, especially if unduly prolonged, does more harm than good (see

STEROID DRUGS). In these cases the use of anti-inflammatory drugs may be justified. These drugs include the non-steroidal anti-inflammatory drugs (see ANALGESIC DRUGS) and the STEROID DRUGS.

Antimalarial drugs

These are drugs used to prevent and treat malaria. The most commonly used preventive drugs are chloroquine (Avolclor, Nivaquine), proguanil (Paludrine), a pyrimethamine and dapsone combination (Maloprim) and mefloquine (Lariam). Chloroquine, quinine and amodiaquine are used in treatment.

Antimetabolites

See ANTICANCER DRUGS.

Antimitotic drugs

See ANTICANCER DRUGS.

Antimycotic drugs

See ANTIFUNGAL DRUGS.

Antineoplastic drugs

See ANTICANCER DRUGS.

Anti-oestrogen drugs

These are drugs that oppose the action of the female sex hormone oestrogen. The most important of these drugs is currently tamoxifen, which antagonizes the action of oestrogens at the tissue receptors. Anti-oestrogen drugs are used to assist in the treatment of breast cancer and to stimulate egg production (ovulation) in infertile women. Side effects of anti-oestrogen drugs include hot flushes, itching of the vulva, nausea, vomiting, fluid retention and sometimes vaginal bleeding.

Antioxidants

Antioxidants are substances capable of preventing the damaging oxidation of organic molecules. Scientists are increasingly recognizing that the ultimate damage to cells and tissues occurring in the course of many disease processes is an oxidation reaction. Oxidation is the process involved in burning, rusting and various other damaging reactions. It is believed, for instance, that the low density lipoproteins that carry cholesterol and other fats to the arteries are capable of causing the deadly disease of atherosclerosis only after they have been oxidized. The oxidation process is brought about by highly active atoms and small chemical groups called oxygen free radicals, and these are capable of starting highly destructive chain reactions in cell membranes and other organic structures. Free radicals are caused by many agencies including:

- radiation
- smoking
- poisons
- infecting organisms
- drugs
- many natural disease processes

Antioxidants are substances that can neutralize or 'mop up' free radicals. The most important appear to be vitamin C, which is water-soluble, and vitamin E, which is fat-soluble. Vitamin E copes mainly with free radicals attacking cell membranes, and vitamin C with free radicals inside and outside cells.

Many well-organized trials have shown that large doses of vitamin C and moderate doses of vitamin E can reduce the risk of a range of important diseases. There is a growing body of opinion that systematic use of antioxidants, for the prevention of disease, is justified.

Anti-Parkinsonism drugs

Parkinsonism is a distressing disorder featuring tremor, poor muscle coordination, stiffness and difficulty in walking. So far there is no cure, but drugs used to control the effects include levodopa (Sinemet), amantadine (Symmetrel), bromocriptine (Parlodel) and selegilene (Eldepryl).

Antiperspirants

These are substances used to reduce the rate of sweating in certain areas of the body where the sweat glands produce sweat that is especially likely to cause body odour. The sweat glands that do this are called apocrine glands and occur mainly in the armpits (axillae) and groins. The sweat from apocrine glands contains not only salty water but also organic material derived from the glands themselves. This material is broken down by bacteria to form odorous substances.

Antiperspirants have an astringent action, narrowing or obstructing the outlet of the sweat glands. Used in excess they may cause skin irritation. Common antiperspirants are alum, aluminium chloride and aluminium chlorohydrate. They are often combined with perfumes.

Antipruritic drugs

These are substances that relieve itching. Calamine lotions or creams are safe and popular, but sometimes more powerful remedies are required, such as local anaesthetics or local ANTIHISTAMINE DRUGS. Both of these are liable to cause skin sensitization and are not much approved of by dermatologists. Antihistamines are sometimes given by mouth for itching. Crotamiton (trade name – Eurax) is often prescribed.

Antipsychotic drugs

Antipsychotic drugs are drugs used to treat the major mental illnesses such as the various forms of schizophrenia, manic depressive illness, mania and severe depression. They are also used to control the behaviour of people who are seriously agitated or aggressive. The drug treatment of psychosis has revolutionized psychiatry and has greatly reduced the number of people confined in mental hospitals.

The most commonly used antipsychotic drugs are the phenothiazine derivatives such as chlorpromazine (Largactil), flupenthixol (Depixol), pimozide (Orap), thioridazine (Melleril) and promazine (Sparine). Lithium is valuable in the management of mania and manic-depressive illness. Most of these drugs act by blocking the action of the nerve stimulator (neurotransmitter) dopamine. Lithium is believed to cut down the production of another neurotransmitter, norepinephrine.

These powerful drugs have side effects, some of which are distressing. Most of them can cause:

- regular jerky movements of some part of the body (dyskinesia)
- lethargy
- drowsiness
- dryness of the mouth
- blurred vision
- difficulty in passing urine

Lithium must be given in very carefully regulated dosage, and toxic effects are common. These include:

- tremor
- staggering
- jerking of the eyes (nystagmus)
- difficulty in speaking
- seizures

Antipyretic drugs

These are drugs which lower raised body temperature. In fever, the body's thermostat is temporarily set at a higher then normal level, so you feel cold and shivering occurs to increase body heat to the required level. Antipyretic drugs work by resetting the thermostat to a normal level. The use of drugs for this purpose is now much less popular than it was prior to the introduction of antibiotics. Nowadays more attention is rightly devoted to removing the cause of the fever – usually infection. The commonest antipyretic drugs are acetylsalicylic acid (Aspirin) for adults and paracetamol for children.

Antirabies serum

This is serum containing antibodies against rabies. It is used to try to prevent the development of the disease in those who have been bitten by a rabid animal. Antirabies serum is combined with the use of a vaccine, given in six injections on days 0, 3, 7, 14, 30 and 90 after the bite.

Antirheumatic drugs

Rheumatism is a general term covering a number of joint disorders featuring inflammation, especially rheumatoid arthritis and osteoarthritis. Many drugs are used to treat rheumatism. Simple ANALGESIC DRUGS are helpful in most cases but may be insufficient. The non-steroidal anti-inflammatory drugs (see ANALGESIC DRUGS) are commonly used. Drugs such as paracetamol and the narcotic analgesic drugs may be useful in relieving pain, but have no anti-inflammatory action.

Rheumatoid arthritis and associated conditions are caused by a disorder of the body's immune system which leads it to attacks its own tissues. The most powerful antirheumatic drugs operate by interfering with the functioning of the immune system and these include the STEROID DRUGS and other IMMUNOSUPPRESSIVE DRUGS. Rheumatoid arthritis is often treated with penicillamine (not to be confused with the ANTIBIOTIC DRUG penicillin), gold, hydroxychloro-quine and chloroquine.

All the major antirheumatic drugs may produce serious side effects. These include:

- kidney damage (penicillamine and gold)
- loss of function of the central part of the retinas causing severe loss of vision (chloroquine)
- osteoporosis, reactivation of latent infections, reduced resistance to new infections (steroids)

Large-dosage steroids may also lead to severe shock in the event of injury or other major illness.

Antiseptics

These are mildly antibacterial substances, usually applied to the skin in the form of solutions, to try to reduce the chances of infec-tion. They are of limited value and are no substitute for thorough washing and cleansing. Alcohol, iodine, hexachlorophane (Phisohex), cetrimide (Cetavlon), allantoin and coal tar (Alphosyl), benzalkonium, thiomersal (Thimerosal) and hydrogen peroxide are among the many substances used as skin antiseptics.

Antiserum

Antiserum is animal blood serum, usually from a horse, which contains useful immunoglobulins (antibodies) to organisms with which the animal has been deliberately infected or to the toxins produced by these organisms (antitoxins). Such serum can be life-saving but can also cause severe reactions. It is usually given by injection into a muscle, and the danger of a severe allergic reaction (anaphylactic shock) is ever present in the mind of the doctor, who will first give a very small test dose just under the skin. Sera are used for the treatment of conditions such as diphtheria, tetanus, rabies, chickenpox and shingles, and Lassa fever.

A range of different antisera is used in medical laboratories to identify unknown organisms. Visible clumping of the organisms will occur when the right serum is added.

Antispasm drugs

Spasm is a tight contraction of voluntary or involuntary (smooth) muscle in any part of the body. Smooth muscle spasm affects especially the wall of the intestine or the bladder. Antispasm drugs act by blocking the action of the nerve activator (neurotransmitter) acetylcholine, which is released from the nerve endings that stimulate the muscle contraction. They are useful in the treatment of bowel colic, as in the irritable bowel syndrome, and in bladder spasm in cystitis and other conditions. Antispasmodic drugs are ANTICHOLINERGIC DRUGS.

Antitoxin

See ANTISERUM.

Antitussive drugs

These are drugs that prevent or relieve cough. Most of them include codeine (Benylin, Dimotane Co, Phensedyl, Terpoin), antihistamines or dextromethorphan (Actifed, Benylin, Lotussin, Sudafed). These drugs work, at a nervous system level, by actually suppressing the cough reflex to the presence of irritating material in the bronchial tubes. As this is one of the body's protective reactions, it is not always a good idea to suppress a cough. But there are some coughs that do little good and seem to go on for ever. So long as your doctor is satisfied that there is nothing seriously wrong, an antitussive medicine can be a great comfort.

Antivenins

A range of specific ANTIDOTES for the bites of venomous animals such as snakes, centipedes, spiders and scorpions. Antivenins are held by doctors in areas in which venomous bites are common. Identification of the animal concerned is important. They are prepared by injecting small and increasing doses of the venom into animals, such as horses, so that antibodies will be produced with specific action against the venom. Such antibodies neutralize the venoms and are called antivenins.

Antiviral drugs

For many years after the introduction of the antibiotics it seemed unlikely that a comparable group of drugs with action against viruses would ever be developed. Viruses are fundamentally different from bacteria and other larger organisms in that they can only reproduce and survive within living cells. It is thus very difficult to find a drug capable of destroying viruses which is not also liable to destroy the host cell.

There have been no fundamental breakthroughs in antiviral treatment, but there have been many small advances based on the rapid growth of knowledge of the biochemistry and genetics of viruses. The most successful approaches, to date, have exploited ways of interfering with the copying (replication) of the virus's genetic material DNA or RNA (ribonucleic acid). This can be done by blocking the chemical activators (polymerase enzymes) that bring about replication. Early drugs, acting on these principles were idoxuridine (Herplex), trifluridine, vidarabine and acyclovir. These drugs are all active against the herpes viruses and the latter, in particular, has had a great success. It is, at the time of writing, the most useful antiviral drug available and has saved many lives in immunocompromised people with widespread herpes infections, as well as preventing an immense amount of pain and distress in people with genital herpes infections and shingles.

The success of acyclovir has encouraged the development of similar drugs such as ganciclovir (DHPG) which is more active against the human cytomegalovirus, and zidovudine (AZT) which has some useful action in suppressing the replication of the AIDS virus, HIV. Unfortunately, AZT is toxic and affects blood production in the bone marrow. Anaemia usually appears after about six weeks of treatment, especially in people with AIDS (the acquired immune deficiency syndrome). Some patients also develop painful muscles.

Some viruses, including the AIDS virus, HIV, make use of an enzyme, reverse transcriptase, to make the necessary second strand of the double helix (RNA viruses have a *single-strand* genetic system). This enzyme has been closely studied by workers hoping to be able to block its action, because any drug capable of doing this would stop the reproduction of the virus concerned. The substances dideoxycytidine and phosphonoformate (foscarnet) are able to do this. Foscarnet can also inhibit the polymerases of all herpes viruses, but it too is toxic.

Ribavirin, acting in a different way, interferes with the replication of a range of viruses including many dangerous respiratory viruses for which effective drugs are badly needed. Some experimental success has been achieved, using the drug in aerosols, against some influenza strains and in serious respiratory syncytial virus infections in children and in Lassa fever. Amantadine and rimantadine are useful against Influenza A virus.

Interferons are substances produced by cells as part of the natural defence against virus infections. They do not act directly against viruses but modify other cells so that they become less capable of cooperating with viruses in achieving the assembly of their components and their replication. Genetic engineering techniques (recombinant DNA) have enabled us to produce enough interferons for clinical trials and limited clinical use, and results are encouraging. The common cold can be treated by direct application to the nose lining, but there are side effects and the treatment is still uneconomically expensive. Genital warts and hepatitis B have been successfully treated.

We are only at the beginning of a process which, if current expectations are realised, may parallel the remarkable advances achieved in the development of the antibiotics in the last fifty years.

Anxiety

See ANTIANXIETY DRUGS, BENZODIAZEPINE DRUGS.

Appetite excess

See APPETITE SUPPRESSANT DRUGS.

Appetite suppressant drugs

These are drugs used to reduce the urge to eat and to help in the control of obesity. On the whole, doctors are not too keen on drug treatment for obesity and usually try to persuade patients to establish new eating habits without the help of drugs. But for many, this is so difficult, and obesity is such a serious health hazard, that they eventually resort to these drugs under close supervision. Drugs, are, however, no substitute for strict calorie counting. Amphetamine and amphetamine-like drugs have a powerful appetite-suppressant effect but are not now used for this purpose. One currently-recommended drug is dexfenfluramine (Adifax). This acts by stimulating the release of the nerve activator (neurotransmitter) serotonin, and has fewer amphetamine-like effects than other appetite suppressants. Other drugs used include diethylpropion (Apisate, Tenuate Dospan), fenfluramine (Ponderax) and phentermine (Duromine, Ionamin). It is unwise to use such drugs for longer than about three months. People with a history of alcohol or drug abuse should avoid them. If there has not been substantial weight loss in this time, the scheme of treatment has clearly failed to reduce the food intake sufficiently. People with a severe weight problem also need plenty of sympathy.

Artery-narrowing drugs

See VASOCONSTRICTOR DRUGS.

Artery-widening drugs

See NITRATE AND NITRITE DRUGS, ANGIOTENSIN CONVERTING ENZYME INHIBITORS, CALCIUM CHANNEL BLOCKERS.

Arthritis

Arthritis is inflammation of one or more joints and may vary considerably in severity. There are several different kinds, the commonest being osteoarthritis, rheumatoid arthritis and gout. These have different features and may require different treatment. Drugs are used to try to control the progress of arthritis and to alleviate the symptoms. Treatment is usually started with NON-STEROIDAL ANTI-INFLAMMATORY DRUGS. These kill pain and damp down inflammation, and the two effects strengthen (potentiate) one another. Very severely affected joints may be treated by local injections of STEROID DRUGS. To try to control the progress of rheumatoid arthritis gold salts, penicillamine, sulphasalazine and chloroquine may be used. Long-term corticosteroid drugs are avoided unless the inflammation is so severe that it cannot be controlled by less powerful drugs.

Gout is treated with colchicine, which can suppress symptoms over long periods, and with the drug allopurinol (Zyloric, Caplenal), which interferes with the formation of uric acid in the body. Uric acid crystals in the joints cause gout. See also ANTIRHEUMATIC DRUGS.

Asthma

Asthma is a potentially dangerous condition. You must be able to judge the severity of your own condition and recognize the need for action. You should understand the effects of different treatments and know the difference between short term, quick relief, drugs which simply combat the immediate narrowing of your bronchial tubes, and longer-acting preventive drugs which reduce the likelihood or severity of attacks. You need a plan for coping with a worsening situation and should clearly understand that if an attack doesn't respond to a bronchodilator inhaler, you probably require steroids. And you must understand that if, in spite of everything, your asthma is going out of control, you are in an emergency situation and require urgent medical attention, day or night.

The best way to take drugs for asthma is by inhalation. This way, they get to the place where they are wanted in the smallest dose needed to produce the desired effect, and with the least chance of causing general upset. Inhalers convert the drug into an aerosol of particles small enough to reach the right place. These may be liquid or a dry powder. Breath-activated powder delivery systems may be easier to use. Lots of asthma patients don't know how to use an inhaler properly. Make sure that you do, because the effectiveness of the treatment depends on it. Read the instructions carefully and follow them exactly or the drug may not get down to the affected bronchial muscles.

Short-term treatment is by drugs like salbutamol (Cyclocaps, Salbulin, Ventide, Ventolin), terbutaline (Bricanyl, Bricanyl SA) and fenoterol (Berotec, Duovent), which stimulate certain of the adrenaline receptors in your bronchial muscles and relax them, so allowing the air to pass freely. If attacks go on in spite of this, you need a mast cell membrane stabilizer to stop your mast cells producing the substances that are causing your bronchial tubes to go into spasm. The best one is sodium cromoglycate (Intal). This cannot stop an established attack, and only works in cases of allergic asthma. Also, the drug must be present in your body when you encounter the pollens, dust, mites, or whatever it is that is causing your asthma. So this is a long-term form of treatment. Sodium cromoglycate is inhaled as a powder, from a 'spinhaler' or an aerosol and should be continued for at least several weeks, as directed by your doctor. If Intal fails, you probably need a steroid such as beclomethasone (Becotide) or betamethasone (Bextasol). These, too, are taken by inhaler, so as to minimize dosage and general effects.

Salbutamol will usually cope with flare-ups, but severe relapses generally require steroids in larger doses and these must be taken by mouth. So don't delay in consulting your doctor. Above all, you should, at all times, know about the state of your bronchial tubes. Ideally, you should be regularly checking, with a peak flow rate meter, the peak rates at which you can breath out. You should be keeping a record of the results, and should know at what point your peak flow rate has become dangerously low.

Athlete's foot

See ANTIFUNGAL DRUGS.

Barbiturates

The class of sedative drugs, formerly used in enormous quantities, but now largely replaced by the BENZODIAZEPINE DRUGS. The best known barbiturates are phenobarbitone (Luminal), amylobarbitone (Amytal), butobarbitone (Soneryl) and thiopentone (Pentothal). Apart from phenobarbitone for epilepsy and pentothal for the induction of general anaesthesia, they are now largely out of fashion and have acquired the same slightly disreputable quality, in medical circles, as the once equally highly regarded AMPHETAMINE DRUGS. Much the same thing is now beginning to happen to the benzodiazepines, which are no longer considered non-addictive and entirely safe.

The origin of the term 'barbiturate' is on a par with the name of the benzodiazepine 'Mogadon' (which is said to have been tested on 'moggies'). Johann Friedrich Wilhelm Baeyer (1835-1917), the Nobel Prize winner, who was working on new derivatives of urea, a constituent of urine, is claimed to have obtained the supplies of urea from which he synthesized the new compound, from a Munich waitress called Barbara. So Barbara's uric acid became barbituric acid. The rest is history.

Barbiturates can cause arthritis, allergic reactions, liver damage and addiction. Their effect can be dangerously increased by alcohol and reduce the effects of various other drugs such as chlorpromazine (Largactil), steroids, phenytoin (Epanutin) and coumarin (see ANTICOAGULANT DRUGS).

Benzodiazepine drugs

The benzodiazepines are sedative and tranquillizing drugs of the Valium, Librium and Mogadon type. They were introduced in 1960 by Hoffman-La Roche whose profits from this group alone have been astronomical. Compared with earlier sedatives, the benzodiazepines are remarkably safe and death from overdose is almost unheard of. In small doses the benzodiazepines relax muscles and relieve anxiety; in larger doses they put people to sleep. They are prescribed and consumed by the billion, about 2 per cent of the population of the Western world taking them regularly to promote sleep, reduce anxiety and relieve depression.

There is no question that they abolish much distress of mind. It is surprising, however, that so little concern has been expressed over the inevitable dependence which must occur when one relies on a drug rather than on one's own resources. Dependence of this sort is not a property of any one particular drug, and the claim that any such drugs are not habit-forming is at least dubious.

This group of drugs includes nitrazepam (Mogadon) and flurazepam (Dalmane) both of which have a prolonged action which may be cumulative; and temazepam (Euhypnos), which has a shorter action and no hangover effect; and diazepam (Valium), chlordiazepoxide (Librium), lorazepam (Ativan), medazepam (Nobrium) and clorazepate (Tranxene), all of which are widely used for the relief of mild anxiety.

Beta-blocker drugs

The term 'beta-blocker' is an abbreviation of 'beta-adrenoreceptor blocking agent'. The adrenoreceptors come in two main classes, alpha and beta, and in several subclasses. The beta receptors are tiny areas scattered all over the heart, the arteries, muscles and elsewhere at which adrenaline and related hormones act. When these hormones contact the receptors their effect is to speed up the heart and constrict blood vessels, so increasing the blood pressure; to reduce the digestive processes; and to widen the airway tubes in the lungs. All this happens in moments of stress and need for action. The beta-blocker drugs have the same general chemical (molecular) shape as the adrenaline molecule and so fit into the receptor sites in the same way, effectively blocking them so that adrenaline, although present, cannot act.

If you have angina, an irregular heartbeat, high blood pressure (hypertension) or a tendency to overreact to stress, the result can be very advantageous. But these drugs could be disastrous for anyone with a tendency to asthma, as they can induce a severe asthmatic attack.

Many beta-blockers have been developed, some with a greater action on one part of the body than on another. Their generic names usually end in '-olol'. The most commonly used beta-blockers include propranolol (Inderal, Beta-Prograne), atenolol (Beta-Adalat, Tenormin), labetalol (Trandate), oxprenolol (Trasicor) and acebutolol (Sectral).

One of the earliest beta-blockers, practolol, was marketed in 1970 after the most stringent tests. Four years later, after many thousands of patients had used the drug, an alert eye specialist noted that he was seeing patients with a most unusual form of dry eye, in which the outer layer of the cornea (the epithelium) was coming off in shreds. All these patients were taking practolol and some became blind. Soon it was found that the drug was also affecting the skin, the inner ear and the inner lining of the abdomen (the peritoneum). Only a small proportion of people on the drug were affected and some kind of immunological process was clearly involved. The drug was withdrawn, except for special cases, and the manufacturer accepted moral responsibility and paid compensation. Beta-blockers in current use have no such effects.

Beta-lactam antibiotics

This is a group of drugs that includes the penicillins and the cephalosporins. All have a 4-member beta-lactam ring as part of the basic structure. Beta-lactam antibiotics function by interfering with the growth of a layer in the cell walls of bacteria that protects them from the environment. Without this layer the bacteria burst open and are destroyed. Human cell walls do not have this layer; this is why these antibiotics are so safe. Bacteria protect themselves against these antibiotics by producing enzymes, beta-lactamases, that block this interference.

Biguanide drugs

Drugs such as metformin and phenformin used to treat maturity-onset (Type II) diabetes. They are part of the group of oral hypoglycaemic drugs. Biguanides act by reducing the efficiency of transfer of charged dissolved substances (ions) across cell membranes thus interfering with the production of glucose by the liver and reducing the energy yield from glucose used as fuel.

Bleeding after surgery

See ANTIFIBRINOLYSIS.

Blocked nose

See DECONGESTANT DRUGS.

Blood clot-dissolving drugs

See TISSUE PLASMINOGEN ACTIVATORS.

Blood clotting, prevention of

See ANTICOAGULANT DRUGS.

Blood clot breakdown

See ANTIFIBRINOLYSIS.

Body bulk control

See ANABOLIC STEROIDS.

Body odour

See ANTIPERSPIRANTS, DEODORIZING DRUGS.

Body fluid excess

See OEDEMA.

Breast cancer

See ANTI-OESTROGEN DRUGS.

Breathing, drugs to stimulate

See ANALEPTIC DRUGS.

Butyrophenone drugs

A group of PHENOTHIAZINE DERIVATIVE DRUGS used in the treatment of schizophrenia. They act as dopamine receptor antagonists. The group includes HALOPERIDOL, triperidol and benperidol.

Calcium channel blocker drugs

Calcium is necessary for the contraction of muscles, and charged atoms of calcium (calcium ions) must pass through special ion channels in the membrane of cells if the muscles are to contract. Calcium channel blockers block this movement and so interfere with the action of the muscle fibres, relaxing the smooth muscle in the walls of arteries so that the blood pressure is reduced and the blood flow through the arteries is improved. This is especially important in the case of the coronary arteries that supply the constantly active heart muscle with blood. Calcium channel blockers are valuable in angina pectoris and in reducing the oxygen consumption of the heart. Like many others, these drugs are broken down in the liver. About four hours after a dose, half the drug has gone.

Nifedipine (Adalat) and diltiazem (Tildiem) are valuable in cases of spasm of the coronary arteries and can relieve angina. They are often used in conjunction with BETA-BLOCKER DRUGS. Verapamil (Cordilox), lidoflazine (Clinium) and prenylamine (Synadrine) are also helpful in cases of irregular heartbeat (cardiac arrhythmias).

These drugs do have side effects including headaches, flushing, fluid retention (oedema), undue slowing of the heart, heart block, and low blood pressure.

Cancer

See ANTICANCER DRUGS, VINCA ALKALOIDS.

Catarrh

See MUCOLYTIC DRUGS.

Cephalosporin antibiotic drugs

See ANTIBIOTIC DRUGS.

Cholesterol-lowering drugs

Constant high levels of fats (lipids), such as cholesterol, in the blood are associated, among other factors, with a raised tendency to the serious arterial disease of atherosclerosis. Atherosclerosis features raised fatty areas (plaques) inside the arteries on which blood clots can form that can close off the artery altogether. This is how heart attacks, strokes and gangrene of the limbs occur. Lipid-lowering drugs are given in certain cases to reduce high levels of fats in the blood.

Most doctors now agree that there is no place for the use of lipid-lowering drugs in people whose high blood cholesterol levels are simply the result of an unhealthy, high-fat diet. Such drugs are no substitute for lots of green vegetables, fruit, fish, skinless chicken, skimmed milk, wholegrain bread and fibre. There are some people, however, for whom they are especially valuable. These are people whose high blood lipid levels are a feature of a genetic disorder known as familial hyperlipidaemia.

These drugs work in different ways. Most of the body cholesterol is synthesized in the liver, and some drugs interfere with the chemical activators (enzymes) which do this. Others interfere with the absorption of cholesterol-containing bile salts from the intestine. They do this by binding to the cholesterol to form an unabsorbable compound that is lost in the faeces. Very large amounts of cholesterol come down the bile duct into the intestine every day but most of this is reabsorbed into the blood with the food. Low levels of bile salts in the blood prompts the liver to convert more cholesterol into bile. Lipid-lowering drugs include cholestyramine (Questran A), clofibrate (Atromid-S) and probucol (Lurselle). There is increasing evidence that it is harmful to lower the blood cholesterol unduly. The side effects of lipid-lowering drugs include diarrhoea, nausea and an increased tendency to form gallstones.

Cold sores

See HERPES.

Cold remedies

It is well known in medical circles that if a cold is left untreated, it lasts for about a week, but that if cold 'remedies' are taken, it will last for about seven days. Jokes of this kind are merely a reflection of the fact that no practical or reasonably economical remedy exists which has any significant effect on most of the two hundred or so regularly mutating strains of viruses that cause the common cold. Some, the rhinoviruses, can probably be controlled by a large daily dose of alpha$_2$-interferon, given as a nasal spray, but this is very expensive and causes nosebleeds.

Millions of pounds are spent every year on over-the-counter common cold remedies, but in spite of implied claims, none of these has anything but a symptomatic effect. There are drugs which stop the nose running and make it easier to breath, drugs which relieve the discomfort of the sore throat, even drugs which make you feel that a cold isn't such a bad thing after all, but these are merely covering up the symptoms and the cold will still be there until the immune system gets the better of it.

Colic in adults

See ANTICHOLINERGIC DRUGS, ANTISPASM DRUGS.

Common cold

See COLD REMEDIES.

Constipation

See LAXATIVES.

Contraceptive drugs

Oral contraceptive pills contain sex hormones in various combinations – the oestrogens ethinyloestradiol and 3-methyl ethinyloestradiol (mestranol) and one of the five progesterone-like substances (progestogens) norethindrone, norethindrone acetate, norethynodrel, norgestrel and laevonorgestrel. Some contain progestogen alone. The oestrogen dosage is very small these days, but the pills are just as effective as the earlier high-oestrogen formulations.

Contraceptive pills work in different ways. Oestrogens prevent ovulation but if this does occur and the egg is fertilized they also interfere with implantation. This means that their action can be, like that of IUDs, somewhat more than purely contraceptive. Progestogens, on the other hand, act on the mucus in the canal of the cervix to keep it thick and viscous and offer a barrier to sperm movement. So their action is more like that of a condom.

Contraceptive pills are highly effective. Recorded failure rates range from one pregnancy per 1000 woman per year to one per 100 woman years. Either way, no one need worry and the method can be considered completely successful in preventing conception. If you forget to take a pill at the usual time you should take one as soon as you remember and you should take the next one at the normal time. But you should realize that if you are 12 hours or more late, the pill may not work and you will be at risk for seven days. If the seven days would take you past you end of the current pill pack you should start another pack straight away.

The pill has a number of side benefits apart from peace of mind and carefree intercourse:

- premenstrual tension (PMT) is often reduced
- periods become regular and less painful
- the likelihood of fibroids of the womb and ovarian cysts and cancers is reduced
- less blood is lost in menstruation
- anaemia is less likely
- the incidence of salpingitis – inflammation of the Fallopian tubes – is reduced

Unfortunately, there is a negative side. Statistically, oral contraceptives slightly increase the chances of cancer of the cervix, but reduce the chances of cancer of the womb lining (endometrium) or of the ovaries. The risk of breast cancer is not thought to be affected. Oral contraceptives do, however, increase the blood-clotting tendency and there is a somewhat higher incidence of deep vein and arterial thrombosis. You will be at greatest risk, in this respect, if you smoke and suffer from severe migraine. Contraceptive pills can also cause:

- weight gain
- breast tenderness
- an increased tendency to acne
- occasional emotional upset
- a sense of fatigue

They have no permanent effect on fertility.

Spermicides, in spite of the name, don't usually kill sperms; they work by making sperms tired so that they can't swim far enough to reach or penetrate the egg. They come in the form of foams, jellies, creams, pessaries and impregnated sponges. The latter can be left in place for about a day and still retain their efficiency. Spermicides actually reduce the chances of acquiring a sexually transmitted disease. They are active against some viruses and probably reduce the chances of getting cancer of the cervix. See also PROGESTOGEN DRUGS.

Coronary thrombosis
See TISSUE PLASMINOGEN ACTIVATORS.

Corticosteroid drugs
See STEROIDS.

Cough
See ANTITUSSIVE DRUGS.

Cramps
Night-time leg cramps are a plague to many people. It now seems likely that the cause is an undue excitability of the millions of tiny connections between the motor nerves and the muscle fibres. The drug quinine bisulphate is often highly effective in reducing this sensitivity. It is taken at bedtime for two weeks and this sometimes provides permanent relief. In other cases the course has to be repeated.

Decongestant drugs
These are drugs used to shrink the congested and swollen lining of

the nose and so relieve 'stuffiness'. Decongestant drugs act on the alpha adrenoreceptors (see BETA-BLOCKER DRUGS) in the small blood vessels of the nose, stimulating them to narrow the vessels supplying the mucous membrane. The result is that less fluid flows into the membrane and it becomes less swollen. You can take these drugs as drops, inhalants or sprays. Drugs used as decongestants include ephedrine (CAM, Franol), phenylephrine, tramazoline (Dexa-Rhinaspray), oxymetazoline (Afrazine) and xylometazoline (Otrivine). Most of these drugs have an adrenaline-like effect (see SYMPATHOMIMETIC DRUGS). Amphetamine was once a popular inhalant decongestant but it aroused too much enthusiasm and was discontinued.

Many decongestants are highly effective in relieving nasal obstruction and reducing the thickness of the mucous membrane. Unfortunately, they have the disadvantage that this effect soon wears off and is followed by 'rebound' recongestion. Inevitably they are overused so that adrenaline- or amphetamine-like effects may be experienced – fast pulse, shakiness and physical and mental overactivity.

Friar's balsam is a long-established decongestant medication. It is a tincture of benzoin, made by dissolving crushed benzoin, aloes, tolu balsam and storax in alcohol. It is popular as an inhalant and has an impressive smell. But the ritual, although hallowed by tradition, is unsupported by evidence of any real therapeutic value.

See also COLD REMEDIES.

Deodorizing drugs

Drugs used to eliminate, mask or prevent undesirable odours. Body deodorants are often ANTIPERSPIRANT DRUGS combined with masking perfumes and have little real deodorant action. They work by reducing the amount of apocrine sweat available for bacterial breakdown – the cause of the body odour. Real deodorants are highly porous substances, such as the clay Fuller's earth, silica gel or activated charcoal and are highly effective, but are unsuitable for general use on the body.

Antiseptics may deodorize by eliminating odour-producing organisms. Hexachlorophene, a powerful germicide, was, at one time, widely used in deodorants. Unfortunately, it was found to cause nervous system damage and is no longer used for this purpose.

Depression

See ANTIDEPRESSANT DRUGS.

Designer drugs

These disreputable substances are modifications of existing psychoactive drugs made so as to produce seemingly new drugs not covered by prohibitive legislation. Designer drugs are produced in secret laboratories for profit and with cynical disregard for their medical and social dangers.

Diabetes

See ANTIDIABETIC DRUGS.

Diarrhoea

For diarrhoea in adults see ANTIDIARRHOEAL DRUGS. Diarrhoea in babies is potentially serious. Because of the ever-present risk of dehydration, diarrhoea in babies should never be taken lightly. Although breast-fed babies are less likely to suffer intestinal infection – the main cause of diarrhoea – than those on the bottle, remember that they normally pass very soft stools. This need cause no concern. But if the faeces are very watery and runny and if there is any sign of general upset, such as fever, vomiting or failure to feed, then medical attention is urgently required. Babies with gastro-enteritis can go downhill very rapidly and you are never justified in delaying definitive treatment while trying over-the-counter remedies.

Diarrhoea in babies can also be caused by lactose intolerance due to deficiency of lactase, the chemical activator (enzyme) which splits disaccharides. Unsplit disaccharides remain in the bowel and retain fluid, causing diarrhoea, distention of the abdomen, bowel noises and failure to thrive. The problem may arise if sugar is added to the feed or if too much, or too concentrated, fruit juice is given.

All babies with diarrhoea require careful attention and you should seek medical advice if the there is any sign of general upset.

Dihydrofolate reductase inhibitors

This is a group of drugs that interfere with the conversion of folic acid to its active form in the body. The effect of this is to interfere with the synthesis of the genetic material DNA. This can be useful in the treatment of leukaemias, cancers, rheumatoid arthritis and the skin disease psoriasis. This group of drugs includes pyrimethamine, trimethoprim, triamterene and methotrexate. When such drugs are necessary, folate deficiency is treated with folinic acid rather than folic acid. Methotrexate potentiates the effects of other dihydrofolate reductase inhibitors.

Diphtheria

This is now so rare that there is a danger young mothers, unaware of how serious the condition is, may neglect to have their babies immunized. Diphtheria is a deadly disease that can be completely prevented by routine immunization. See also ANTISERUM.

Diuretic drugs

Various heart, kidney and liver disorders can cause water to accumulate abnormally in the tissue spaces of the body, or within some of the body cavities. Fluid in the tissues is called oedema and fluid in the cavities is called an effusion. Tissue fluid accumulation is worst in the lower parts of the body – the ankles and lower back and the lower parts of the lungs. Oedema can interfere with body function – especially in the lungs – and causes unwanted weight gain and other disadvantages. It is always an indication that something is wrong. If possible, the cause should be corrected. Usually, correction of the cause will clear up the oedema, but it is often necessary to get rid of the excess fluid in a more direct manner. This is the job of the diuretic drugs. Normally, the kidneys filter very large volumes of water out of the blood. If all this water entered the urine, we would quickly die of dehydration, so most of it is reabsorbed back into the blood. Diuretics act on certain parts of the kidneys to prevent some of this reabsorption of water and allow a proportion of it to pass out in the urine. When they do this, the blood becomes concentrated and the excess fluid in the tissues is drawn into it, thus relieving the oedema.

Diuretics are very effective. Frusemide (Lasix) or bumetanide (Burinex) act within an hour and the effect on the kidneys lasts for about six hours. Large quantities of urine may be produced – up to 10 litres in a day. Too rapid loss of fluid may reduce the blood volume undesirably and can be dangerous. There may also be danger from the undue loss of potassium from the body, but doctors are aware of this danger and, if necessary, give potassium tablets to make up losses. Thiazide diuretics, such as bendrofluazide (Aprinox) or hydrochlorothiazide (Esidrex, Hydrosaluric) produce a smaller output of urine spread over a longer period.

Diuretics are nearly always taken by mouth, but sometimes, in an emergency, they may be given by injection. In long-term conditions causing oedema they are given in a dosage just sufficient to keep the fluid from accumulating in the tissues.

In addition to those mentioned, diuretic drugs include spironolactone (Aldactone), acetazolamide (Diamox), ethacrynic acid (Edecrine), amiloride (Moduretic, Midamor) and cyclopenthiazide (Navidrex). These drugs act in slightly different ways on the kidneys, but they all have the same useful effect.

Side effects of diuretic drugs include:

- damage to hearing (frusemide and ethacrynic acid)
- muscle pain (bumetanide)
- stomach and duodenal ulcers (spironalactone)
- painful enlargement of the breasts in men (spironalactone)
- impotence (bendrofluazide, hydrochlorothiazide, cyclopenthiazide)
- loss of potassium (all except 'potassium-sparing' diuretics such as amiloride (Moduretic), triamterene, spironolactone)

Potassium loss can cause vomiting, diarrhoea, muscle stiffness, muscle weakness, drowsiness, apathy, loss of memory, excess urine production and thirst. Severe potassium loss can cause sudden stoppage of the heart (cardiac arrest). Excess of potassium is equally dangerous and this occasionally happens when a potassium-sparing diuretic is used.

Dopamine receptor agonists

These are drugs that have an effect on the body similar to that of dopamine, and roughly similar to that of ADRENALINE. They include bromocriptine and lysuride and are used to treat Parkinson's disease, acromegaly, overproduction of the hormone prolactin, and to suppress or prevent milk secretion. Possible side effects include nausea, vomiting, constipation and unwanted fertility in women.

Dopamine receptor antagonists

Drugs that compete with dopamine to occupy and block the dopamine receptor sites in the body. They include butyrophenones and thioxanthenes used to treat psychosis. Possible side effects include those of the PHENOTHIAZINE DERIVATIVE DRUGS, especially chlorpromazine.

Drugs of abuse

See PSYCHOACTIVE DRUGS.

Duodenal ulcer

See ANTACID DRUGS, PROTON PUMP INHIBITOR DRUGS.

Dyspepsia

See ANTACID DRUGS.

Emetic drugs

Emetics are drugs which induce vomiting. They are little used nowadays, but are sometimes valuable in the treatment of poisoning and in the re-conditioning treatment of alcoholism. Ipecacuanha (Alophen) and apomorphine are the most commonly used.

Endometriosis
See PROGESTOGEN DRUGS.

Epilepsy
See ANTICONVULSANT DRUGS.

Female sex hormones
See OESTROGEN DRUGS.

Fever
See ANTIPYRETIC DRUGS.

Fibrinolytic drugs
This is a group of drugs capable of breaking down the protein fibrin which is the main constituent of blood clots. They are thus able to disperse dangerous blood clots (thromboses) that have formed within the circulation. They include streptokinase, alteplase, anistreplase and urokinase. Possible side effects include bleeding at needle puncture sites, headache, backache, tiny blood spots in the skin (purpura) and allergic reactions.

Filariasis
See ANTHELMINTIC DRUGS.

Fits
See ANTICONVULSANT DRUGS.

Fluid-removing drugs
See DIURETIC DRUGS.

Fluid retention
See DIURETIC DRUGS.

Free radicals
See ANTIOXIDANTS.

Fungus infections

See ANTIFUNGAL DRUGS.

Germs

See ANTISEPTICS, ANTIBIOTIC DRUGS.

Glucosidase inhibitor drugs

Glucosidase is a chemical activator (enzyme) that takes part in the breakdown of complex sugars such as starches and glycogen. A glucosidase inhibitor is a drug that interferes with this action so that sugars are much less easily absorbed into the body from the intestine. They are known as 'starch blockers' and are helpful in bringing about weight loss in people with Type II diabetes. Unfortunately, the excess of complex carbohydrates in the intestine tends to cause flatulence. The real answer, of course, is to eat less of them.

H$_2$ receptor antagonists

See ANTACID DRUGS.

Hallucinogenic drugs

These are drugs that induce hallucinations. Most of them are derived from plants such as the desert peyote cactus, *Lophophora williamsii* from which mescaline is derived, the psilocybin-containing 'sacred mushrooms' and the seeds of the morning glory flower, which contain lysergic acid. These drugs can precipitate an acute psychotic illness in predisposed people. At one time they were used by some psychiatrists to investigate or to try to treat mental illness but few now believe they are of any medical value.

Hangover

A hangover is the state of physical and mental distress experienced on waking after an evening of overindulgence in alcohol. The symptoms are not caused exclusively by the ethanol (ethyl alcohol). This drug is certainly toxic to the brain and highly irritating to the stomach lining, but it is difficult to have an alcoholic binge without taking in more than just ethanol. The alcohol and aldehyde congeners which help to give character to alcoholic drinks are also toxic.

Heavy drinkers are also likely to spend most of the evening in an atmosphere of dense smoke, eating little or nothing and, as a result, possibly developing low blood sugar (hypoglycaemia). It is difficult to separate all the different causes of the morning after misery. The headache is not caused by ethyl alcohol, almost all of which will have been metabolized before the headache starts. The seat of the pain is the arteries of the scalp and the brain coverings (the meninges). The brain itself is insensitive to pain. Acetaldehyde is probably the chief culprit, but the problem is not helped by loss of sleep and by the dehydration resulting from the diuretic effect of the alcohol.

Alcohols act on the receptors for the neurotransmitter gamma aminobutyric acid (GABA), affecting nerve function in a way that many scientists believe is responsible for the behavioural changes characteristic of inebriation. Adaptation to this effect can readily be acquired by those who really try, and some of the features of the hangover are undoubtedly related to withdrawal. This is why the 'hair of the dog' is so welcome and effective, and why chronic alcoholism is so common. Little can be done to avoid hangover, once the poison has gone down. Only measures which reduce the rate of absorption of alcohol – slow drinking of long drinks, taken with plenty to eat, are likely to be of any value. PAINKILLING DRUGS are of some value, but, as in so many other cases, prevention is better than cure.

Hay fever

'Hay fever' is not a particularly accurate term. The condition is not associated with fever, nor is it particularly associated with hay. The experts call it 'seasonal allergic rhinitis' or 'pollinosis' and it probably affects 2% of the population. It affects the sexes equally and is commonest between the ages of 15 and 25. Atmospheric pollen has decreased markedly in the last 30 years, but, unfortunately, pollutants have increased sixfold in that time. It seems likely that oxides of sulphur and nitrogen and increased lower atmosphere ozone concentrations, to say nothing of tobacco smoke, have caused respiratory tract damage, allowing readier access of pollens to the immune system.

Rhinitis is simply inflammation of the nose lining and this is not necessarily allergic nor related to seasonal factors as in the case of hay fever. Non-seasonal allergic rhinitis is due to many causes such as house dusts, house dust mites, or animal fur or skin flakes, and commonly occurs all the year round. Both seasonal and non-seasonal allergic rhinitis affects people with a hereditary tendency to atopy – a condition featuring childhood eczema and asthma. People with atopy are hypersensitive to substances which are harmless to 80% of the population. These substances are called 'allergens' and they may be eaten or inhaled and cause many problems.

In hay fever the allergens are the seasonal pollens in the inhaled air. The spring type of seasonal allergy is caused by airborne tree pollens, especially elm, birch elder, oak and maple, and the summer type is due to grass and weed pollens. Sometimes the problem is caused by airborne fungus spores, usually in a localized geographic area. Pollen grains enter the noses of the sufferers where they are trapped by a layer of sticky nasal mucus. Lysozyme enzymes then digest off the outer coat and release the protein allergens. Situated within and just under the epithelial lining of the nose are millions of mast cells. These granule-filled cells are of fundamental importance in allergy, for the granules contain highly active substances including histamine, proteases, prostaglandin D2 and a range of leukotrienes. These have many effects when released: they contract smooth muscle, including that in the walls of the bronchioles, increase the leakage of fluid from small veins so that membranes swell, stimulate mucus and watery secretion from the nose lining and cause local itching and burning. The leukotrienes are even more potent narrowers of the air tubes – bronchoconstrictors – than histamine. The proteases (protein-splitting enzymes) are thought to be capable of damaging small blood vessels.

In people with allergic rhinitis, a previous exposure to the allergen has resulted in the production of the antibody immunoglubulin E (IgE) and the mast cell membranes already have the IgE in place. This so sensitizes the mast cells that whenever they are triggered by the same allergen they immediately start leaking out their powerful contents. The result, of course, is the general misery of the hay fever victim.

The most effective measure is to avoid the allergen, and this may even involve changing residence, using air filters or masks, keeping bedroom and car windows closed (especially on motorways), avoiding areas known to be major sources of the pollen and avoiding going out in the early evening when pollen grains which have been carried up during the day begin to fall again.

Symptomatic treatment is valuable and is the commonest response to the problem. ANTIHISTAMINE DRUGS block the receptor sites for histamine and can be quite effective. The H1 antagonists terfenadine and astemizole have no detectable sedative or antispasm effects. Terfenadine is probably the antihistamine of choice. Cromoglycate (Cromolyn) has a more immediate effect and is said to operate by blocking the reaction of the allergen with the mast cell membrane, but it cannot deal with symptoms due to histamine and prostaglandins already released. It is commonly used in the form of a nasal aerosol. DECONGESTANT DRUGS are also helpful and can, to some extent, counteract the sleepiness caused by antihistamines. They are best given by mouth, as the nasal spray preparations lead to rebound congestion. Beclomethasone-type STEROID DRUGS are extremely effective and, used locally, do not seem to interfere with adrenal gland function.

Heart attack
See TISSUE PLASMINOGEN ACTIVATORS.

Heart disease
See CALCIUM CHANNEL BLOCKER DRUGS.

Heart irregularity
See ANTIARRYTHMIA DRUGS.

Heart pain
See ARTERY-WIDENING DRUGS.

Herpes

Herpes is caused by the herpes simplex virus. There are two strains, herpes simplex virus, type 1, often called HSV-1, which causes herpes around the mouth and nostrils, and HSV-2, which causes genital herpes. The herpes viruses seem to prefer to live inside nerve tissue and for most of the time, they remain dormant in the nerves, causing no trouble. This is a safe place, from their point of view, and it is almost impossible to get rid of them.

Every now and then, dormant viruses become active, reproducing rapidly, moving to the skin and causing the well-known itching, tingling discomfort and spreading clusters of painful little crusting blisters. We don't know, for certain, why the dormant viruses flare up, but they often do so during a feverish illness, or at times of stress or emotional upset or after exposure to bright sunlight. Some people get an attack after taking certain foodstuffs or drugs. It is probable that the fighting strength of the viruses is kept under control most of the time by the immune system and that herpes only flares when the immune system is coping with demands elsewhere. People whose immune systems are deficient, as in AIDS, have a very bad time with herpes, which often spreads to parts of the body not normally affected.

The trouble with trying to treat herpes is that, because the drugs act to stop the viruses reproducing, we don't ever know when is the right time to start. Unfortunately, before each flare-up, reproduction has gone on quietly for quite a while, so there are always plenty of viruses around before we start thinking of treatment. So, short of treating all the time, the idea is to start treatment at the earliest possible moment. The first suggestion of a tingle is the signal for getting on with it.

There are several drugs with action against the herpes virus. These include Vidarabine (Vira-A), Idoxuridine (Herpid) and acyclovir (Zovirax). Of these, acyclovir is the safest and most effective and has largely replaced the others. It works well, not only for the herpes viruses, but also for the closely similar varicella-zoster virus which causes shingles and chicken pox. Acyclovir is a remarkable drug which remains practically inert until it hits herpes viruses. These contain an enzyme which converts the acyclovir to the active form, acyclovir triphosphate, and it is this which stops the virus DNA from reproducing.

Acyclovir can safely be taken by mouth and it is widely distributed throughout the body. It is excreted in the urine and about half the dose has gone in three hours. It is also available as a cream for the treatment of herpes on the lips and eyes. Genital herpes is best treated by the tablets, for the use of the cream may encourage resistant strains of the virus to emerge. The dose will be prescribed by your doctor and you should on no account try to economize. Large doses are used for primary attacks, but, unfortunately, do not eradicate the infection. If you suffer severe recurrent herpes you can dramatically reduce the frequency and severity of the attacks by taking a tablet three times a day. Don't treat yourself without medical advice. See also ANTI-VIRAL DRUGS.

High blood cholesterol

See CHOLESTEROL-LOWERING DRUGS.

High blood pressure

You can't afford to ignore raised blood pressure because its complications cause more deaths and severe disability than any other group of diseases. Coronary thrombosis and stroke – the two major killers of the Western world – are the major risks, but raised blood pressure can also severely damage your heart, kidneys and eyes. Unfortunately, high blood pressure does not produce symptoms unless it is severe or has already reached a fairly advanced stage and has caused damage to the blood vessels and the heart. So it has to be looked for. Every adult should have regular checks. Remember that proper and effective treatment can largely eliminate the additional risk of these serious complications.

If you have moderately raised blood pressure, and are a fairly typical middle-aged person, you must not expect to be able to carry on with your accustomed lifestyle and think that the problem will be solved just by taking a pill twice a day. You are probably overweight and taking very little exercise. You may be living a risky, stressful life. Perhaps you smoke cigarettes. If treatment is to be successful, you are going to have to modify your lifestyle. Smoking is deadly and must be cut out. Even the most otherwise effective drug treatment may fail to reduce the probability of death if you continue to smoke. Changing your eating habits will not be easy, but this, too, is important. In many cases, the change to a healthy, natural lifestyle, with regular exercise, little food, no smoking, and perhaps a reduction in salt intake, will be sufficient, in itself, to get your blood pressure down to normal. Regular attendance at your doctor's, for check-ups, will give you confidence and help to reduce stress levels.

Your doctor has a wide range of effective drugs at his or her command (see ANTIHYPERTENSIVE DRUGS, ANGIOTENSIN CONVERTING ENZYME INHIBITORS), but also has difficult and complex decisions to make. Among others, there is the decision whether to use drugs at all. Your body may have adapted to raised blood pressure, so reducing it may actually cause you, for a time, to feel worse, rather than better. Until you readjust to a normal level, you may feel weak and lacking in energy. You may feel depressed and find you have a tendency to dizziness or faintness on standing up. It is important to bear these possibilities in mind. Your doctor has to take them into account and to make sure that you do not use these symptoms as reasons for avoiding treatment. The idea is to try to get your blood pressure down with the minimum possible dosage of drugs, and, in this, your lifestyle really matters. See also BETA-BLOCKER DRUGS.

Hives (urticaria)

See ANTIHISTAMINE DRUGS.

HMG-CoA reductase inhibitors

These are drugs that interfere with the synthesis of cholesterol by the liver and are used to reduce abnormally high blood cholesterol levels. They include lovastatin, simvastatin and pravastatin. Possible side effects include muscle disorder with pain and weakness, liver damage, insomnia, headache, nausea, dyspepsia, diarrhoea and abdominal cramps.

Hookworms

See ANTHELMINTIC DRUGS.

Hormone replacement therapy (HRT)

See OESTROGEN DRUGS.

Hydrophobia

See ANTIRABIES SERUM, ANTISERUM.

Hypertension

See ANTIHYPERTENSIVE DRUGS.

Hypnotic drugs

These are drugs that help you to sleep. They are also called sedatives or soporifics. Hypnotics damp down the action of the whole nervous system and especially that of the surface (cortex) of the brain – the seat of consciousness. Overdosage is always dangerous and causes:

- coma
- interference with normal breathing
- reduced blood pressure
- a drop in body temperature
- abolition of normal reflex activity

Long-term use of hypnotic drugs makes you more tolerant to their effects. It also leads to addiction with withdrawal symptoms. Because of this long-term use of these drugs is now generally deprecated by doctors. Hypnotic drugs are potentially dangerous to life and are often used in suicide attempts. They include chloral hydrate, bromide salts and BARBITURATES, none of which are now commonly used, and the BENZODIAZEPINE DRUGS, which are used in great quantity. Chloral hydrate is still sometimes used to sedate sleepless children, but ANTIHISTAMINE DRUGS, which also have a sedative effect, are more commonly given for this purpose.

The automatic prescription of hypnotic drugs in response to a complaint of insomnia is bad medicine. It is necessary to take time to analyze the cause of the insomnia and deal with it directly. If hypnotics are used at all, they should be used sparingly and only for short periods. Millions of people are addicted to hypnotic drugs.

Hypoglycaemics, oral

See ANTIDIABETIC DRUGS.

Imidazole drugs

A class of antifungal and antibacterial drugs effective against a wide range of bacteria and fungi. The group includes METRONIDAZOLE (Flagyl), MEBENDAZOLE, THIABENDAZOLE, CLOTRIMAZOLE (Canesten), ketoconazole and MICONAZOLE.

Indigestion

See ANTACID DRUGS.

Infection

See ANTIBIOTIC DRUGS, ANTISEPTICS.

Inflammation

See ANTI-INFLAMMATORY DRUGS, STEROID DRUGS.

Insomnia

The first thing to say is that sleep-inducing drugs are not the mainstay of the treatment of insomnia. They are prescribed in great quantity, mainly because doctors don't have enough time to go into the real reasons for the insomnia. But you do have the time, and you should look very closely at the real nature of your sleep problem. Consider, first, whether you are having difficulty in falling asleep or whether the difficulty is in staying asleep.

If the former, consider whether your problem could be due to anxiety or tension, so that you just lie awake for ages, unable to relax and allow yourself to drift off to sleep. Perhaps you have had too much coffee or tea in the evening. Caffeine will certainly keep you awake and alert. Business, personal, marital or other worries may be the cause of your tension. If so, they are likely to seem insoluble, especially when you are lying awake in bed, but the proper approach is to try to resolve these problems, and meantime to put them right out of your mind, not to take sleeping pills. When the difficulty is in getting off to sleep, you will probably sleep well enough once you have succeeded in relaxing properly.

If you fall asleep easily enough, but wake repeatedly, try to analyze the cause. Could it be that you are so exhausted that you go to bed too early, and then naturally awake in the early morning, having had enough sleep? Are you sedating yourself with alcohol every night? This gets you off to sleep quite well, but the effect is often short-lived and early waking is common. Are you depressed? This is a common cause of interrupted and restless sleep and often features early waking. Are you in pain? Are you trying to give up sleeping tablets to which you have acquired tolerance?

When the insomnia is clearly due to any such cause, the right treatment is to deal with the cause. If you go to bed exhausted, perhaps you need a short nap in the middle of the day. This can be invaluable. Half an hour can make all the difference and can improve your afternoon performance and leave you fresher in the evenings. Depression caused by external misfortune or bereavement will nearly always pass in time, but some depressions require proper treatment (see ANTIDEPRESSANT DRUGS). Pain, of course, should be fully investigated and the cause removed, if possible. If this cannot be done, the right approach is to give effective painkillers (ANALGESIC DRUGS), supplemented, if necessary, by sleeping pills, given for short periods only.

If you suffer persistent insomnia for no obvious reason, or if you are going through a very difficult period, but can see light at the end of the tunnel, there may be justification for the use of HYPNOTIC DRUGS, given in the hope that you may, thereby, get back into the habit of normal sleeping. But taking sleeping pills over long periods is bad medicine. You are likely to become addicted and eventually suffer withdrawal problems. You will probably become tolerant and have to increase the dose steadily to get the same effect. Also, the kind of sleep induced in this way is neither natural nor properly refreshing.

If you must have hypnotics, the benzodiazepine drugs, like Mogadon or Noctamid are to be preferred to barbiturates like Amytal or Soneryl. The diazepines, which include the longer-acting Valium and Librium, are safer than the barbiturates, but are still liable to cause physical dependence. Avoid them all, if you can.

Irritable bowel syndrome

See ANTICHOLINERGIC DRUGS, ANTISPASMODIC DRUGS.

Itching

See ANTIPRURITIC DRUGS.

Jock itch

See ANTIFUNGAL DRUGS.

Lassa fever

See ANTISERUM.

Laxatives

The subject of constipation is of enduring interest to mankind as well as of enormous commercial importance to the pharmaceutical industry. Like many subjects of wide popular interest, however, it is fraught with fallacy. There is a general belief that some calamity will befall anyone who fails to empty his or her bowels at least once a day. This belief is without foundation. Some people have a satisfying bowel motion three times a day, others three times a week. Some feel the need to go even less often. So long as the passage is easy, without undue straining, and with a satisfying sense of completeness, all these patterns are normal.

Constipation can certainly cause symptoms but these are not, as is alleged by many alternative medicine practitioners, the result of the absorption of 'toxins' from the bowel. These symptoms can be produced by packing the rectum with sterile cotton wool. Constipation does not cause halitosis, distention, abdominal discomfort, belching or headache.

Constipation is as often imaginary as real, and many people, who believe that a daily bowel action is essential to health, severely abuse their lower intestines with laxatives, suppositories and enemas. This response to an imaginary disorder can produce a real one. Anxious, fastidious people, especially those whose food intake is small, often feel that it is essential to get rid of 'unclean' excreta every day. Some become very anxious if there is no bowel motion. The constant use of laxatives in these circumstances can lead to an irritable bowel disorder. Depressed people often excrete less than average and the awareness may, in turn, make the depression worse.

Constipation is, of course, a symptom and not a disease. It has many causes. These include:

- deliberate suppression of evacuation
- chronic obstruction from tumours or bowel strictures
- painful piles
- various neurological disorders such as Parkinson's disease and spinal cord injuries
- ANTICHOLINERGIC DRUGS such as atropine
- ANALGESIC DRUGS such as codeine
- bismuth salts
- ANTICONVULSANT DRUGS
- ANTIDEPRESSANT DRUGS

Constipation is essentially a disorder of civilized societies and is almost unknown among peoples whose diet is largely vegetable with a high fibre content. Such people produce frequent bulky stools and are free from many of the colonic disorders suffered by those of us who enjoy more expensive diets.

The first step in tackling the constipation syndrome is to ensure adequate bulk in the stools. This is easily done by adjusting the diet so as to replace refined carbohydrate with foods containing much vegetable fibre. Plenty of fruit, vegetables and bran-containing cereals should be taken. The best drug for constipation is bran. This is what is left when flour is extracted from cereals. It contains up to half its weight in cellulose vegetable fibre which has the property of taking up large quantities of water. So bran should always be accompanied by a good fluid intake. It is hard to eat too much bran. This kind of regime will produce bulky, soft stools and regular motions.

When a laxative is required for long-term use, the only form that should be considered is one of the bulking agents. These are safe, act slowly and gently and are not habit-forming. Bran is the best, but most people feel that something more expensive is bound to be better and go in for nicely packaged preparations of methyl cellulose, which is much the same, apart from the price. Isogel is made from psyllium seeds and contains mucilage which, like bran cellulose and methyl cellulose, also swells and bulks up with water.

Other forms of laxative, safe for occasional use, include wetting agents such as Dioctyl and Poloxamer 188, lubricants such as liquid paraffin, and osmotic agents like Lactulose or Epsom, Glauber or Rochelle salts. These agents are not absorbed, but remain in the bowel, retaining and attracting water and thereby increasing the bulk of the stools. Plenty of water should be drunk with all of these. Avoid irritant laxatives, like castor oil, senna, cascara, and so on. These should never be used on a regular basis. Enemas may be needed if you are ill or debilitated, but should be used under medical supervision. Colonic irrigation should probably be regarded as a rather dubious recreational activity.

Leukaemia

See DIHYDROFOLATE REDUCTASE INHIBITORS.

Malaria

See ANTIMALARIAL DRUGS.

Manic-depressive illness

See ANTIPSYCHOTIC DRUGS.

Maturity onset diabetes

See BIGUANIDE DRUGS, SULPHONYLUREA DRUGS.

Menstrual excess

See PROGESTOGEN DRUGS.

Menstruation, painful

See PERIOD PAINS.

Mental disorders

See ANTIPSYCHOTIC DRUGS, DOPAMINE RECEPTOR ANTAGONISTS, PHENO-THIAZINE DERIVATIVE DRUGS.

Migraine

See SEROTONIN ANTAGONIST DRUGS.

Monoamine oxidase inhibitors

See ANTIDEPRESSANT DRUGS.

Motion sickness

This is the effect, on susceptible people, of exposure to persistent sustained movement, whether in a car, aircraft, boat, train, swing, flight simulator or space-craft. It may also occur when people are subjected to any unusual motion or even to the sight of an apparently moving horizon. The word 'nausea' comes from the Greek word *naus*, meaning a 'ship', so the problem has been around for a while.

After a variable period of exposure to the unaccustomed motion, the victim begins to feel uneasy and this progresses rapidly to severe distress. There is yawning, overbreathing, increased salivation, nausea, abdominal discomfort, pallor, sweating of the face and hands, headache, and vomiting. Air-swallowing, dizziness and an intense sense of fatigue may also occur. If the motion continues, these symptoms persist for several days, often progressing to apathy, depression, total loss of appetite and sometimes loss of the will to live.

The cause of motion sickness is uncertain, but it is known to be related to overstimulation of the balancing mechanism in the inner ears. It does not occur when these, or the acoustic nerves, have been destroyed. The information your brain needs for orientation in space comes from your balance mechanism, eyes and the nerve endings in your joints, muscles and skin. These three sources reinforce each other and can compensate for each other's deficiencies. In motion sickness there seems to be a mismatch between the three stabilizing systems.

Psychological factors and the state of the environment are also relevant. You are more likely to be sick in a stuffy or malodorous enclosure than in the fresh air, and a full stomach does not associate well with a heaving vertical motion. To some extent travel sickness is a conditioned reflex; people who expect to be sick often become so the moment they perceive motion.

Since motion sickness is related to a sustained loss of any fixed base by which to judge bodily position, it is helped if you can fix your eyes on some unmoving point or line, such as the horizon. This is another reason to get up on deck. Other measures claimed to be helpful include a steady draught of fresh air, sitting with your head tilted backwards, and taking frequent small meals.

The best drug treatment for motion sickness is small doses of whichever drug you have found, by experience, to be most effective. Useful drugs include atropine (Belladonna) and its derivative hyoscine, and antihistamine drugs with atropine-like action, such as cyclizine (Diconal), promethazine (Avomine, Phenergan) or dimenhydrinate (Dramamine). You must take one of these drugs at least an hour before the motion starts, for once the vomiting has started, tablets or capsules may be rejected. Also, these drugs take a little time to act. All effective anti-motion sickness drugs have a sedative effect and you should never take them along with alcohol. Like all ANTICHOLINERGIC DRUGS they may also cause dry mouth and may blur the vision. Longer-acting drugs like promethazine or meclozine may be started up to a day before the journey begins. Be very careful to avoid overdosage, especially in children, by repeating the dose too frequently.

Mucolytic drugs

These are drugs which make mucus more liquid and less sticky. They are used most to assist in the coughing up of sputum, but are occasionally used for other purposes where excess mucus is a problem. The most commonly used mucolytic drug is acetylcysteine (Parvolex, Airbron).

Mucus excess

See MUCOLYTIC DRUGS.

Multivitamin preparations

These are combinations of vitamins, most of which are purchased and consumed by people who have no need for them and derive no benefit from them. People on normal diets do not suffer from vitamin deficiency unless they are suffering from a rare malabsorption disorder. Vitamins A and D are dangerous if taken in excess. Hypervitaminosis A and D are well-recognized clinical syndromes. All the B vitamins are co-enzymes and are needed for many of the chemical reactions of the body. But the amounts required are very small and are adequately provided by all but extremely inadequate or grossly unbalanced diets. Any taken in excess of the requirements are wasted. The amounts of vitamin C in multivitamin preparations are quite inadequate if they are being taken as ANTIOXIDANT DRUGS; at least 1000 mg a day are required for this purpose. Vitamin E, taken as an antioxidant, should be taken separately in a dose of about 400 mg for an adult. Large doses of vitamin E are dangerous for babies.

Muscarinic antagonists

This group of drugs opposes the action of acetylcholine (see ANTI-CHOLINERGIC DRUGS) and is used to treat certain cases of urinary frequency and incontinence.

Muscle-relaxant drugs

Anaesthetists commonly use drugs, such as tubocurarine (Curare), pancuronium, gallamine and suxamethonium (Scoline) to paralyse muscles and allow safer anaesthesia. In more general use are some drugs which reduce spasm of voluntary muscles without affecting voluntary movements. These may be useful in nervous system diseases, such as stroke and cerebral palsy, which cause the muscles to go into spasm, and in rheumatic and other diseases featuring painful sustained contraction of muscles. These drugs include baclofen (Lioresal), which is a derivative of one of the body's nerve activators (neurotransmitters) (GABA), and dantrolene (Dantrium) which acts directly on the muscles.

Other muscle-relaxing drugs are diazepam (Valium), chlormezanone (Trancopal), carisoprodol (Carisoma) and methocarbamol (Robaxin).

Muscle spasm

See ANTICHOLINERGIC DRUGS, ANTISPASMODIC DRUGS, MUSCLE-RELAXANT DRUGS.

Narcotic drugs

See ANALGESIC DRUGS.

Nausea

See ANTIEMETIC DRUGS.

Nervous system stimulants

See ANALEPTIC DRUGS.

Nitrate and nitrite drugs

The action of these drugs is to relax the circular layers of smooth muscle in the walls of arteries. The effect of this is that the arteries widen so more blood can flow though. This is called 'vasodilatation'. The nitrates are short-term vasodilators but are valuable in treating angina pectoris, in which the blood flow to the heart muscle is reduced by coronary arteries narrowed by the artery disease atherosclerosis. The nitrates are also of value when the pumping efficiency of the heart is reduced (heart failure).

One of the most commonly used nitrates is nitroglycerine, the explosive, which, for medical purposes, is mixed with inert (inactive) material and made safe. This is best taken in a tablet placed under the tongue from which absorption into the blood is rapid. Amyl nitrite is a volatile liquid supplied in thin-walled glass capsules which must be broken before the liquid can be inhaled. Isosorbide dinitrate (Cedocard), and isosorbide mononitrate (Elatan) are used to try to prevent anginal attacks.

Because they widen many of the arteries in the body, nitrates can cause fainting and collapse by reducing the blood pressure too suddenly and too much. This is likely only if they are taken in excessive dosage or if you have become hypersensitive to them. Nitrates may cause severe headaches by stretching the pain-sensitive tissues around the brain arteries – a kind of drug-induced migraine.

NSAIDs

Non-steroidal anti-inflammatory drugs. See ANALGESIC DRUGS, ANTI-INFLAMMATORY DRUGS.

Obesity

See APPETITE SUPPRESSANT DRUGS.

Oedema

Certain disorders, especially of the heart, kidneys or liver, may cause water to accumulate abnormally in the tissue spaces of your body or even within your abdomen. This is called oedema. At first, there is just an increase in weight, but later your ankles and the lower parts of your trunk may swell up. The swelling tends to affect the dependent parts of your body, so if you are lying down, it may affect your back. The swelling is different from ordinary fat accumulation. If you press it firmly with your fingers you leave hollow pits which slowly flatten as the displaced fluid returns. Sometimes oedema makes your face puffy.

Oedema usually indicates, either that your heart is not pumping the blood back from your tissues fast enough or that there is not enough protein in your blood to draw the water out of the tissues. Severe oedema often also affects the lungs, where fluid may accumulate, making your breathing less efficient. Your doctor, listening to the bottoms of your lungs with a stethoscope, may hear the faint crackling noise made by fluid in the air sacs. The oedema fluid is mainly water, but it contains quite a lot of salt and this tends to keep it in the tissues. Reducing salt in your diet will often relieve oedema.

Oedema is always an indication of some other disorder and your doctor will want to treat the cause. Often, this will clear up the oedema, but, for the sake of your comfort and to improve the function of your organs, it may be necessary to get rid of the excess fluid in a more direct manner. This is where the DIURETIC DRUGS come in. Diuretics can be highly effective. A dose of furosemide (Lasix) or Burinex acts within an hour and has an effect on the kidneys lasting for about six hours. Large quantities of urine may be produced – as much as 10 litres in a day. There can be dangers from too rapid loss of fluid and the blood volume can be reduced to undesirable levels. There may also be danger from the undue loss of potassium from your body, but your doctor will see that you come to no harm from these causes. You may be given potassium tablets to make up losses. Sometimes, in an emergency, a diuretic drug may be given by injection, but usually they are taken by mouth. In a persistent condition they are given in a dosage just sufficient to keep the fluid from accumulating in the tissues.

Oestrogen drugs

The oestrogens are a group of steroid female sex hormones secreted mainly by the ovaries, but also by the testicles. Oestrogens bring about the development of the female secondary sexual characteristics. In conjunction with progesterone, they act, each month in the non-pregnant, to prepare the lining of the womb for implantation of the fertilized egg (ovum). They have some anabolic properties (see ANABOLIC STEROIDS).

Oestrogen drugs are substances chemically related to the natural hormones. They include oestradiol, ethinyloestradiol, mestranol and diethylstilboestrol. They can be given by mouth, by implants under the skin, by vaginal pessaries and by skin patches. They are used to treat inadequate ovary function. They are the basis of hormone replacement therapy (HRT) for menopausal symptoms and to limit postmenopausal osteoporosis. They are used to stop milk production (lactation) and to treat widespread cancers of the prostate gland. Most of all, they are used as oral contraceptives (see CONTRACEPTIVE DRUGS).

Oestrogen therapy rarely produces serious complications, but it may be complicated by a number of possible side effects. These include:

- nausea and vomiting
- weight gain
- bloating due to water retention
- painful breasts
- increased blood clotting with a higher risk of thrombosis
- gall stones
- high blood pressure

Oestrogens given as hormone replacement therapy may increase the risk of cancer of the womb and may encourage the growth of any existing breast cancer. Some experts believe that the addition of progesterone eliminates the risk of womb cancer. You should be sure that no breast tumour is present before starting HRT.

Opium derivatives

Crude opium as a solution in alcohol, known, expressively, as laudanum was once the only major narcotic ANALGESIC DRUG and was widely used for all sorts of appropriate, and inappropriate, purposes. Purified preparations containing a mixture of the many opium alkaloids are still used. These include Nepenthe, Papaveretum and Omnopon.

The main alkaloid narcotic derived from opium is morphine, and this is still extensively used. It is a valuable drug both for its powerful painkilling property and for the calm euphoria, and relief from shock and anxiety, it gives those who are the victims of severe accidents or other dangerous and painful misfortunes. Heroin (diamorphine) is even more powerful, but has long been banned for medical use in most countries in the world as offering no advantage over morphine except increased solubility. Heroin, still used medically in the UK, is converted into morphine in the body.

In addition to relieving pain and distress of mind, morphine adversely affects breathing, sometimes fatally, stops coughing, promotes sleep, causes vomiting and constipation, and makes the pupils small. Codeine, a mild narcotic analgesic drug is another opium derivative. It is used mainly for relief of moderate pain and to check diarrhoea and irritable, nonproductive coughing.

Oral hypoglycaemic drug,

See ANTIDIABETIC DRUGS.

Osteoarthritis

See ANTIRHEUMATIC DRUGS.

Over-the-counter (OTC) drugs

These are drugs that may be purchased directly from a pharmacist without a doctor's prescription. Current government policy in the UK is to extend the range of OTC drugs. A number have already been de-restricted and this trend is expected to increase. This will place an additional advisory responsibility on pharmacists.

Painkillers

See ANALGESIC DRUGS.

Parkinson's disease

See ANTI-PARKINSONISM DRUGS.

Penicillin antibiotic drugs

See ANTIBIOTIC DRUGS.

Period pains

Period pain is caused by cramping contractions of the womb which interfere with the blood supply to the muscles and other cells and cause them to be slightly damaged. Whenever any cell in the body is damaged, substances called prostaglandins are released from the cells. Prostaglandins have a variety of actions, but the one we are interested in, here, is the pain-stimulating effect. Injected prosta-glandins cause severe headache and pain in the blood vessels.

The common pain relievers – Aspirin and ibuprofen – are similar in their action. These drugs block the production of prostaglandins by damaged cells, and this is how they relieve pain. Drugs like morphine act on the brain; others act on nerve conduction. But the Aspirin-like drugs act directly on damaged cells and work solely by preventing the production of the substances which cause the pain.

The Aspirin-like drugs are powerful and should be treated with respect. Never use ordinary Aspirin, only the soluble variety, and never use Aspirin if you have indigestion or a previous history of ulcer trouble. Sensitivity to Aspirin, especially in people with other allergies, is rare, but can cause alarming and often dangerous reactions, including severe asthma and dangerous swelling inside the Adam's apple. This can obstruct your breathing. So if you have genuine allergies, beware of Aspirin and the Aspirin-like drugs. Polyps in your nose are a special warning of this danger. Remember that such side effects are common to the whole group of Aspirin-like drugs.

The popular painkiller Panadol or Paracetamol, also has its dangers. The drug is broken down in the liver and an overdose can cause liver failure and death, after a few days. There is an antidote, called methionine, but this must be taken early. The safest form is called Pameton, in which paracetamol is combined with the liver-protecting methionine.

Brufen, or ibuprofen has, in the past, been taken primarily for relief of joint pain, but it has other uses and seems to be better than Aspirin for menstrual period pain. It is certainly safer than Aspirin, although it causes tummy upset in about one person in ten. Like Aspirin, it can prolong bleeding time and people, such as asthmatics, sensitive to Aspirin can react to it in exactly the same way. It should be taken very cautiously by people with liver disease.

These drugs are most effective if taken one or two days before menstruation starts and continued for one or two days after the onset of the period. Should they give insufficient relief, try a little codeine as well. If all else fails, you may need to have your ovulation temporarily suppressed by a low-dose, oestrogen-progesterone contraceptive pill. This, of course, is a matter for your doctor.

Perspiration

See ANTIPERSPIRANTS.

Phenothiazine derivative drugs

This is an important group of drugs widely used to treat serious mental (psychotic) illness and to relieve severe nausea and vomiting. Examples are chlorpromazine (Largactil), thioridazine (Melleril) and perphenazine (Fentanyl). See ANTIPSYCHOTIC DRUGS.

Poisoning

See Chapter 6, ANTIDOTE.

Poor blood flow

See NITRATE AND NITRITE DRUGS.

Potassium channel blockers

These drugs close the channels in cell membranes through which potassium ions pass out of cells. The effect of this is to increase the excitability and probability of action of the cells. Potassium channel blockers include the sulphonylurea group of drugs used to treat maturity-onset diabetes. These increase the output of insulin from the beta cells of the Islets of Langerhans in the pancreas.

Potassium channel openers

This group of drugs opens the channels in cell membranes through which potassium ions pass. Efflux of potassium reduces the excitability of the cell so that it is less likely to act. Potassium channel openers include the muscle relaxant drugs minoxidil and hydralazine used to treat high blood pressure.

Progestogen drugs

The progestogen drugs are a group of drugs chemically similar to the natural hormone progesterone. They are used in oral contraceptives (see CONTRACEPTIVE DRUGS, OESTROGEN DRUGS) to help to prevent ovulation and to make the mucus in the cervix less easily penetrable by sperms. They are also used to treat menstrual disorders.

Prostaglandins

Prostaglandins are a group of chemical substances (unsaturated fatty acids) that occur throughout the tissues and fluids of the body. They are produced from fatty substances (phospholipids) in the outer membranes of cells when these are damaged. Released prostaglandins function as hormones. There are quite a number of different prostaglandins with different, often opposing, actions. These include:

- narrowing of arteries
- widening of arteries
- stimulation of pain nerve endings
- clumping of blood particles called platelets to promote blood clotting
- prevention of clumping of blood platelets and reduction of blood clotting
- induction of abortion
- reduction of stomach acid secretion
- relief of asthma

Some painkilling drugs, such as Aspirin, act by preventing the formation of prostaglandins in the injured tissue. Synthetic prostaglandin drugs are used to induce labour, to procure abortion and to relieve stomach and duodenal (peptic) ulcers. They are also used to treat abnormal persistence, after birth, of the fetal duct that bypasses the lungs during life in the womb – the condition known as patent ductus arteriosus. We are still finding out about the prostaglandins.

Proton pump inhibitor drugs

A recently-introduced class of drugs that control the production of stomach acid. The proton pump is the chemical activator (enzyme) hydrogen-potassium ATP-ase. This is involved in the final stage of acid production by the specialized cells of the stomach lining (the parietal cells). A proton pump inhibitor is a drug that blocks the action of this enzyme. So far, the only drug with this action is omeprazole (Losec). This drug can be used in cases in which H2 receptor blocker drugs have failed to reduce acid sufficiently (see ANTACID DRUGS).

Psoriasis

See DIHYDROFOLATE REDUCTASE INHIBITORS.

Psychoactive drugs

These are drugs whose action modifies in some way the state of the mind. They include mental stimulants such as amphetamine, cocaine, caffeine, and nicotine; depressants such as the BENZODI-AZEPINE DRUGS, the BARBITURATES, alcohol, and TRANQUILLIZER DRUGS; the narcotic ANALGESIC DRUGS, such as morphine, pethidine and methadone; and the HALLUCINOGENIC DRUGS, such as LSD, mescaline and psilocybin.

Purgatives

See LAXATIVES.

Pyrazolone drugs

This is a group of non-steroidal anti-inflammatory drugs (NSAIDs) that includes phenylbutazone and azapropazone.

Quinolone drugs

A group of synthetic antibiotic drugs that includes nalidixic acid, ofloxacin and enoxacin. These drugs act by inactivating an enzyme, DNA gyrase, necessary for replication of the organisms. They are often useful for treating infections with organisms that have become resistant to other antibiotics. They are administered by mouth. Possible side effects include nausea, vomiting, diarrhoea and abdominal pain, headache, restlessness and tiredness. Psychiatric disturbances occasionally occur.

Rabies

See ANTIRABIES SERUM, ANTISERUM.

Resistant infections

See QUINOLONE DRUGS.

Retinoid drugs

A class of drugs related to vitamin A that act on the skin to cause drying and peeling and a reduction in oil (sebum) production. These effects can be useful in the treatment of acne, psoriasis, ichthyosis and other skin disorders. They are administered by mouth or applied as a cream. Possible side effects are many and some are serious. They include severe fetal abnormalities (if taken by pregnant women), toxic effects on babies (if taken by breast-feeding mothers), liver and kidney damage, excessive drying, redness and itching of the skin, and muscle pain and stiffness. Trade names are Retin-A and Roaccutane.

Rheumatism

See ANTIRHEUMATIC DRUGS.

Rheumatoid arthritis

See ANTIRHEUMATIC DRUGS, DIHYDROFOLATE REDUCTASE INHIBITORS.

Roundworms

See ANTHELMINTIC DRUGS.

Sadness

See ANTIDEPRESSANT DRUGS.

Salivation

See ANTICHOLINERGIC DRUGS.

Schizophrenia

See ANTIPSYCHOTIC DRUGS.

Sedative drugs

See ANTIANXIETY DRUGS, ANTIEMETIC DRUGS, ANTIPSYCHOTIC DRUGS, BARBI-TURATES, BENZODIAZEPINE DRUGS, BETA-BLOCKER DRUGS, HYPNOTIC DRUGS.

Seizures

See ANTICONVULSANT DRUGS.

Serotonin antagonist drugs

Serotonin, or 5-hydroxytryptamine (5-HT) is an ADRENALINE-like nerve stimulator (neurotransmitter) that has a marked effect on mood and excitability. Serotonin-antagonist drugs oppose the action of this substance and produce a variety of effects, including reduction of depression and the control of migraine. The action is not clearly understood.

Severe pain

See OPIUM DERIVATIVES.

Sexual criminality

See ANTIANDROGEN DRUGS.

Sleeping drugs

See HYPNOTIC DRUGS.

Snake bite

See ANTIVENINS.

Steroids

The group of steroid drugs known as the corticosteroids were first isolated from the outer layer (cortex) of the adrenal gland, where the natural hormone cortisol is produced – hence the name. A steroid is a member of the large chemical group, related to fats, which includes sterols such as cholesterol, bile acids, sex hormones, many drugs and the adrenal cortex hormones. Corticosteroid drugs are chemically similar to the natural steroid hormones.

These drugs have many uses and can be given by injection, by mouth, in the form of ointments or creams or as eye or ear drops. They are highly effective against inflammation, and are prescribed for many conditions in which inflammation may cause damage to the body. These include:

- inflammatory diseases of the bowel, such as regional ileitis (Crohn's disease) and ulcerative colitis
- joint inflammation, such as rheumatoid arthritis
- inflammation of arteries, as in temporal arteritis
- inflammation in the eye (uveitis)
- asthma
- hay fever (allergic rhinitis)
- eczema

The steroids are used to help to suppress the immune responses which lead to the rejection of a donated organ transplant and are often life-saving in conditions of severe stress in which the production of natural hormones is inadequate. And they are given as hormone replacement therapy to people with disease of the adrenal glands (Addison's disease).

It seems to be a law of nature that anything capable of a powerful effect can also do a lot of harm. Powerful drugs nearly always have major side effects and the corticosteroids, given in large dosage, are no exception. But you need to view this with a sense of proportion. Steroid skin ointments and creams, used occasionally, are unlikely to do any harm and, indeed, some steroids for local application are considered so safe that you can buy them over the counter without a doctor's prescription. Powerful steroids used on the skin, however, are liable to cause skin atrophy and thinning. Steroids used in an inhaler are also unlikely to have any significant general side effects, as the dose is very small and, properly used, the drug goes only where it is needed. But steroids in high doses for long periods will inevitably cause some side effects and these vary with the dose and how the drug is given. The more important of these include:

- suppression of the body's production of natural steroids
- reactivation of latent infections

- an increased susceptibility to new infections
- the breakdown of partly-healed stomach or duodenal ulcers
- osteoporosis
- diabetes
- high blood pressure
- excessive hairiness (hirsutism)
- glaucoma
- cataract

Suppression of natural steroid production doesn't matter too much so long as steroid is being taken, but suddenly stopping the treatment is very dangerous. All patients on long-term steroid treatment should carry a card indicating, in detail, the treatment they are having. In the event of a severe accident or other major stress, this knowledge can be life-saving. The risks of side effects of steroids vary considerable from person to person and may be minimal. Doctors, however, will always balance the risks against the risks and disadvantages of not using high-dose, long-term steroids.

The decision to give long-term steroids to young children must be balanced against the fact that these drugs cause severe stunting of growth. It must be remembered that the same effect may be caused by serious childhood illnesses, for which steroids may be needed.

Stimulation

See ANALEPTIC DRUGS.

Stomach ulcer

See ANTACID DRUGS, H$_2$ RECEPTOR ANTAGONIST DRUGS.

Stuffy nose

See DECONGESTANT DRUGS.

Sulphonamide drugs (sulpha drugs)

The sulphonamides, which appeared in the 1930s, were the first effective antibacterial drugs that could safely be taken by mouth.

They were, rightly, hailed as 'wonder drugs' and saved millions of lives by their action against streptococci and staphylococci and other organisms, until they were largely supplanted by the ANTIBIOTIC DRUGS.

Sulphonamides are now used to a limited extent, but are still valuable for urinary infections where their high concentration, as they are excreted from the body, makes them efficient. The combination of the sulphonamide sulphamethoxazole and the folic acid antimetabolite trimethoprim produces the highly successful and widely used drug Septrin. Certain sulphonamides are very poorly absorbed from the intestine and so are useful and safe in treating some intestinal infections.

Sulphonylurea drugs

A class of drugs used in the treatment of maturity onset (Type II), non-insulin dependent diabetes. They are taken by mouth. Also known as oral hypoglycaemic drugs.

Sweating

See ANTICHOLINERGIC DRUGS, ANTIPERSPIRANTS.

Swollen ankles

See DIURETIC DRUGS.

Sympathomimetic drugs

These drugs act on the body to cause effects similar to those of adrenaline or of the sympathetic part of the autonomic nervous system (see ANTICHOLINERGIC DRUGS). These effects are generally stimulating and include:

- increase in the heart rate
- increase in the blood supply to the voluntary muscles
- slowing of digestion
- widening (dilatation) of the pupils of the eyes
- widening of the lung air tubes (bronchial tubes)
- tightening of the muscle rings (sphincters) around the outlet of the bladder and the bowels

These effects are produced by the natural hormones adrenaline and noradrenaline and by drugs such as amphetamine, ephedrine, isoprenaline, methoxamine, salbutamol, phenylephrine, metaproterenol, terbutaline and salmeterol. All these are called sympathomimetic drugs. The effects are complicated by the fact that there are several different receptors for adrenaline-like substances. These are divided into the alpha-adrenergic receptors (alpha-1 and alpha-2) and the beta-adrenergic receptors (beta-1 and beta-2). Some drugs stimulate some of these receptors, but not others. Some stimulate all adrenoreceptors. In general, drugs which block the adrenoreceptors (see BETA-BLOCKER DRUGS) are antagonistic to the sympathomimetic drugs.

Tapeworms

See ANTHELMINTIC DRUGS.

Teething

The time of appearance of the primary (milk) teeth is very variable. Some babies are actually born with one or more teeth, much to the alarm of the breast-feeding mother. Others still have no teeth by one year, again causing alarm. Both extremes are normal and need cause no concern. In most cases, the first teeth – the central incisors (biting teeth) – appear around six to nine the other incisors. Around 10 to 16 months, the first molars (grinding teeth) appear and at 16 to 20 months, the canine (tearing teeth) appear. The second molars usually erupt sometime between the second and third years of life.

Teething causes gum tenderness, some pain, and dribbling, and the baby will spend much time investigating his or her mouth. Teething can certainly lead to fractiousness and crying, but this is seldom a serious problem. Other conditions may cause these symptoms which may be wrongly attributed to teething. Evidence of undue distress should lead to investigation.

Teething powders and chewing rings should be avoided. Aspirin is now out because of Reye's syndrome, but a suitable dose of a paracetamol preparation (Calpol, Junior Disprol, Junior Panaleve) can be a great comfort to all concerned, including the

Wellcome Foundation which claims 70% of the £8.6 million world market. A mild local anaesthetic preparation with an astringent to reduce salivation (Dentinox teething gel) may be helpful.

Tension

See MUSCLE-RELAXANT DRUGS, ANTIANXIETY DRUGS.

Tetanus

See ANTISERUM.

Tetracycline antibiotic drugs

See ANTIBIOTIC DRUGS.

Thiazide diuretic drugs,

See DIURETIC DRUGS.

Thioxanthene drugs,

A group of antipsychotic drugs related to the PHENOTHIAZINE DERIVATIVE DRUGS. The group includes flupenthixol and clopenthixol.

Threadworms

See ANTHELMINTIC DRUGS.

Tinea

See ANTIFUNGAL DRUGS.

Tissue plasminogen activators

A tissue plasminogen activator (TPA) is a naturally occurring chemical activator (enzyme) that can dissolve blood clots. Since so many serious conditions are caused by clotting (thrombosis) within arteries, or the breaking free of clots in veins (see ANTICOAGULANT DRUGS), obviously a substance that can break down clots and restore the blood flow is of major medical importance. Other clot-dissolving enzymes, such as streptokinase and urokinase, have been in use for many years. These have achieved some success if given within an hour or two of the thrombosis. TPA appears to have several major advantages over these earlier drugs. It is believed to be responsible for opening up (recanalizing) blood vessels blocked by thrombosis, and it is much more effective in dealing with mature blood clot – a mass of the protein fibrin – than either streptokinase or urokinase. TPA can be produced by genetic engineering methods and is marketed under the name alteplase (Actilyse, Activase).

Many important studies have now been done on patients with recent coronary thromboses, people with unstable angina and people in whom blood clots have travelled to the lungs causing the dangerous condition of pulmonary embolism. TPA can open up blocked coronary arteries within 19 to 50 minutes after it is injected, restoring the blood supply to the heart muscle. If the affected area of muscle has not been killed, function is restored. TPA can dissolve large clots carried to the lungs from the veins, and it can stop these clots from forming (deep vein thrombosis). The drug does not produce antibodies. The results are uniformly excellent and there is no doubt that TPA is an important advance in treatment.

All this sounds wonderful, but nothing is ever perfect in this world. TPA has one major side effect – a tendency to cause bleeding. Because of this the drug is dangerous in people who have recently had a stroke, in those with any bleeding tendency and in people with a history of stomach or duodenal ulcer. TPA drugs do not, of course, distinguish between an unwanted thrombosis and a naturally occurring sealing plug of clot. So bleeding readily occurs at any point of blood vessel injury such as a recent injection site or at the points of insertion of blood vessel catheters.

Toxocariasis

See ANTHELMINTIC DRUGS.

Tranquillizers

The term 'tranquillizer' is not really scientific but is useful as a grouping for a range of drugs having mild muscle-relaxing and anxiety-relieving action. The major ANTIDEPRESSANT DRUGS and ANTIPSYCHOTIC DRUGS are excluded from this group. So the tranquillizers include such drugs as the BENZODIAZEPINE DRUGS, the BARBITU-RATES, the BETA-BLOCKER DRUGS and some of the mild HYPNOTIC DRUGS. Other drugs such as meprobamate (Equanil) and buspirone (Buspar), are also used.

See also ANTI-ANXIETY DRUGS.

Travel sickness

See MOTION SICKNESS.

Trichomonal vaginitis

See IMIDAZOLE DRUGS.

Tricyclic antidepressant drugs

See ANTIDEPRESSANT DRUGS.

Tricyclic antipsychotic drugs

See ANTIPSYCHOTIC DRUGS.

Urinary incontinence

See ANTICHOLINERGIC DRUGS.

Vasoconstrictor drugs

These are drugs which cause the circular smooth muscle coat in the walls of arteries to contract so that the vessel is narrowed and the rate of blood flow though it reduced. The natural hormones adrenaline and noradrenaline act on particular alpha-adrenergic receptors (see SYMPATHOMIMETIC DRUGS) to cause vasoconstriction.

Both nicotine and cocaine are powerful vasoconstrictors and the former has been implicated in the gangrene-producing disease thromboangiitis obliterans (Buerger's disease).

See also DECONGESTANT DRUGS.

Vasodilator drugs

These are drugs which cause arteries to widen so that the blood flow through them is improved. Vasodilator drugs are often valuable, but sometimes cause alarming effects by lowering the blood pressure too much. They include NITRATE AND NITRITE DRUGS, drugs such as prazocin and hydralazine, and CALCIUM CHANNEL BLOCKER DRUGS such as nifepidine.

Vinca alkaloids,

A group of drugs that interfere with cell division and are of value in the treatment of certain cancers. They are used especially in acute leukaemias and malignant lymphomas. They include vinblastine and vincristine. Possible side effects include:

- inflammation and clotting in veins at the site of injection
- hair loss
- interference with nerve function
- interference with bone marrow blood cell production

Virus infections

See ANTIVIRAL DRUGS.

Vomiting

See ANTIEMETIC DRUGS.

Water retention

See DIURETIC DRUGS.

Weight control

See APPETITE SUPPRESSANT DRUGS.

Wind and colic

Greedy or hungry babies often swallow air along with their feeds and this air becomes compressed by peristalsis and may cause colic, pain and much crying. It often leads to regurgitation of food, much to the annoyance of the person who has to clean up, and may also feel obliged to replace losses. Traditional burping methods help, but many parents will need something more reliable. Dill water, a gentle carminative may be useful, as may dimethicone (Dentinox Colic Drops) which is a silicone polymer oil, useful as a skin barrier cream or ointment base, but used here to reduce surface tension and allow froth bubbles to coalesce so that the air may more easily be expelled from either end.

Worms

See ANTHELMINTIC DRUGS.

4. HOW DRUGS ARE TAKEN

Most drugs are taken by mouth, but there are many other ways in which drugs can get into your body.

Drugs by mouth

These are dispensed as compressed, coated or uncoated, tablets; as cylindrical, two-piece capsules which are slid open to insert the drug in powder or granule form; as sealed gelatin ovoids or 'pearls' containing a liquid; or, rarely, as soft rolled pills or as cachets of rice paper or other material. There is no harm in biting tablets before swallowing, if you can stand the taste. This will speed absorption of the drug. Don't open capsules, or you are sure to lose some medication and might adversely affect the rate at which the drug is absorbed.

Some drugs are absorbed directly from the mouth itself. Nitroglycerine for angina, for instance, acts more rapidly if you put the tablet under your tongue than if you swallow it. Some drugs, such as Aspirin and alcohol, are absorbed from the stomach, but most pass on to the small intestine, which is the normal absorption zone for food.

Drugs likely to cause severe stomach irritation are often dispensed in a capsule made of a material which will not dissolve until it reaches the small intestine. These are called 'enteric-coated' capsules. A wide range of 'slow-release' formulations is available, usually in capsule form containing layers of the drug, or tiny spherules, each coated with a protective covering.

'Three times a day after meals'

Most drugs have to be taken several times a day, and you may be a little uncertain about exactly what a doctor means by 'three times a day' or 'four times a day'. Ideally, the intervals between doses of a drug should be equal, so that a drug to be taken three times a day might be taken at 8 am, 4 pm and midnight. But the prescription might order 'three times a day after meals'. This may seem a little unimaginative on the part of the doctor. A drug to be taken four times a day might thus be taken at 8 am, 2 pm, 8 pm and 2 am. Perhaps a little inconsiderate.

The fact is that for the great majority of drugs, it really isn't necessary for the 24 hours to be mathematically divided in this way. In most cases you can safely spread the doses evenly over the waking day and forget about the alarm clock. Usually, 'three times a day after meals' just means 'after breakfast, lunch and evening meal'. You should, however, clarify this point with your doctor whenever you get a new prescription. There are some cases in which the timing of the doses really does matter.

The question of whether drugs should be taken before, with, or after food can be important. Drugs taken on an empty stomach are most rapidly absorbed into the circulation and have their effect most quickly. This may be what is needed. Drugs taken with or immediately after a meal are diluted by the food and are usually absorbed more slowly. This may be what the doctor wants. He or she may also be concerned that the drug prescribed may be irritating to the empty stomach and may cause nausea or even vomiting. Some drugs, however, are actually changed and made less active by certain foods or drinks, or their absorption into the blood may be interfered with. Such drugs will be ordered to be taken before meals. There is never any objection to your drinking a little water to help the tablet or capsule over the back of your tongue.

Watch the dose

Do take dosage seriously. Some people act on the principle that if a little of something is good for you, a lot must be even better. This is a dangerous idea in relation to drugs. In most cases there is a reasonable leeway between the effective dose and the toxic dose (see pages 20-21), but you would be very ill-advised to rely on this and take it on yourself to increase the dosage of a powerful drug. Take *exactly* the number of tablets or capsules ordered, and in the case of mixtures, use standard spoon sizes. You can get 5 ml plastic spoons from the chemist. These give accurate dosage for fluids. Some mixtures *must* be thoroughly shaken before use. Otherwise, the early doses will be inadequate and the later doses far too strong.

There is more flexibility in the case of some over-the-counter mixtures, but it is a good idea to stick to the recommended dose. Remember, however, that the standard adult dose is assessed for an adult of average weight. This means that if you are much below the average it will be easier for you to take an overdose. Dosage for children (anyone below 12) is even more important and you should follow instructions scrupulously. Don't give adult drugs to children unless this is ordered by a doctor.

Other routes of administration

Drugs may get into you by a surprising variety of routes.

Skin

Drugs are applied to the skin in ointments, creams, lotions, powders or solutions. In general, these drugs act only on the skin and are intended to treat skin disorders. Normally, applied to the intact skin, they are not absorbed in sufficient quantity to have any effect on the rest of your body. There are, however, some dangers you should know about. If the surface of the skin is raw, extensively broken or ulcerated, it is possible for considerable quantities of a drug, applied to such areas, to be absorbed into the bloodstream. So do be careful about overdoing applications of drugs or other local applications to the skin.

Some drugs can be given in patches applied to the skin for slow absorption. This route has been employed for hormone replacement therapy, for contraception, and for other purposes. The idea seems to be becoming more popular.

Injections

Many drugs are given by injection, and this may take various forms. Drugs may be injected *into* the skin, as in a tuberculin test (intradermal injection), under the skin (subcutaneous injection), deeply into a muscle (intramuscular injection) or directly into the blood flowing in a vein (intravenous injection). Drugs given by injection usually act more quickly than drugs taken by mouth. Drugs given intravenously may act within seconds.

The injection route is often necessary because many drugs, if taken by mouth, would be destroyed by the stomach acid or the digestive enzymes. Some drugs are too irritating to be injected subcutaneously or intramuscularly and would cause serious tissue damage if given in this way. These drugs must be given by slow, careful intravenous infusion so that they are gradually diluted as they are carried into the general circulation. Drugs are seldom given into arteries (which carry blood from the heart) unless an arterial catheter is already in place.

'Depot' injections are drugs made up in a medium, often oil or wax, which allows slow release over days or weeks. They may be subcutaneous or intramuscular and the quantity injected is much larger than the normal dose. Many different drugs and hormones may be given in depot form. They include antibiotic drugs, corticosteroid drugs, antipsychotic drugs, sex hormones and contraceptive drugs (see Chapter 3).

Sometimes drugs are given in the form of implants. These are small tablets or other formulations which are buried under the skin through a tiny cut (incision) which is then closed with one or two small stitches. Injections are occasionally given into the bone marrow, into the cerebrospinal fluid surrounding the spinal cord, or into the abdominal cavity.

Drugs by inhalation

Many drugs may be rapidly absorbed into the circulation, or have a local effect, if they are inhaled in an aerosol or as a fine powder. Nicotine from cigarette smoke, for instance, reaches the brain within a few seconds of inhalation. Other drugs are less well absorbed when taken by this route.

Inhalation from various kinds of inhaler is, for instance, an important route of access for drugs used to treat asthma and some other respiratory conditions. The advantage of this route is that it allows drugs to reach the required areas in high concentration, while minimising the effects on the body generally. Thus, steroid drugs can be taken by inhalation with relative safety and with minimal risk of side effects. It is, however, important that you should be sure you are using the inhalers properly. There is something of an art in this if the drug is to get where it should go and not simply be sprayed all over the inside of your mouth. It is all a matter of timing.

Other routes
Drugs can get into the circulation through any absorbent body surface, such as the inner lining of the bowel or vagina. It is often best to give certain drugs in the form of rectal suppositories. These are bullet- or cone-shaped medications moulded from a substance such as cocoa butter, with which the drug is mixed, and which melts at body temperature. They are easily passed in through the anus. Similar vaginal pessaries may be prescribed, usually to treat vaginal infections.

Drugs may also be absorbed from the nose lining, from the conjunctiva of the eyes, or from the inside of the bladder or urine tube (urethra). These routes are usually chosen when limited local drug action is required and are not normally used if full absorption is desired. Cocaine 'snorters' rely on nasal absorption. This causes such extreme constriction of the nasal blood vessels that the mucous membrane lining is sometimes destroyed and a hole appears in the thin wall between the two sides of the nose. A perforation of the nasal septum is, however, one of the more minor dangers of the habit (see Chapter 5).

Points to note

- If you find that a medicine is causing strange effects or making you sick, contact your doctor without delay. Don't just put up with it; you might be having a potentially dangerous reaction.
- If, after a few days, you are sure that the treatment is not having the desired effect, contact your doctor.
- Never stop taking a drug that is working well until you have taken the full prescribed course. To do so is asking for trouble. You might well find that you get worse again *and that the original treatment is no longer effective.*

5. DRUGS OF ABUSE AND DEPENDENCE

Drug abuse is one of the central social problems of the present day, and is a major cause of crime, ill-health and death. It mainly involves young people. At the same time, thousands of elderly people are, in a less dramatic and obvious way, quietly abusing drugs. Young people are using marijuana, cocaine, amphetamine, heroin, LSD, MDMA (ecstasy) and various inhaled volatile substances. Older people are abusing benzodiazepines and barbiturates. People of all ages are abusing alcohol and tobacco.

People who are dependent on a drug are always thinking about it and will get it and take it regardless of consequences. Usually, such people rely for their comfort of mind or body on the repeated use of the drug. In some cases, the addiction is physiological – that is, the use of the drug has led to persistent changes in the way the body functions, so that its absence causes physical symptoms (withdrawal symptoms). In others, the dependence is mental only. A feature of dependence is the loss of control over the taking of the drug and the lengths to which the addict will go to get supplies. Theft or prostitution are common. Well-off people need not necessarily resort to crime to maintain the habit, but would probably do so, if there were no other way.

The term 'drug abuse' is not so easily defined as you might think. The great majority of the inhabitants of the world are habitual drug takers, mainly of caffeine, nicotine and alcohol, and many of them are addicted to these drugs. This kind of indulgence is not generally regarded as 'abuse' and there are many who, likewise, do not consider the occasional use of substances like marijuana or cocaine as abuse. In many parts of the world, drugs, such as betel nut, pan or opium are used habitually, and few of these people would regard themselves as abusing drugs. But no one would deny that there are millions who use alcohol and tobacco to the detriment of their health. There are also millions who, with or without the tacit connivance of doctors, abuse drugs such as Valium or Librium, meprobamate (Equanil) and many others.

So the phrase 'drug abuse' is unclear and unsatisfactory. It has come to mean, in effect, the use of any drug which is currently disapproved of by the majority in a particular society. In an attempt to clarify the concept of drug abuse, drugs used to alter the state of the mind for recreational or pleasure purposes are often divided into 'hard drugs' and 'soft drugs'. The distinction is somewhat arbitrary, but hard drugs are those liable to cause major emotional and physical dependency and thus an alteration in the social functioning of the user. This group includes heroin, morphine, opium and similar natural or synthetic substances. The soft drug group includes tranquillizers, sedatives, cannabis, amphetamines, alcohol, hallucinogens and tobacco. This classification into 'hard' or 'soft' does not indicate that one group is safer than the other. The abuse of 'soft' drugs, such as alcohol and tobacco kills many times more people than abuse of 'hard' drugs.

So the term 'drug abuse' might be more usefully taken to mean the use of a drug in such quantity or frequency as to cause physical, mental or social damage to the user. It's not so much the drug that's being abused as the person who takes it.

Nicotine

This drug is derived from the leaves of the tobacco plants *Nicotiana tabacum* and *Nicotiana rustica*. It is a colourless to amber oil with a strong smell of tobacco and an intensely bitter taste. Nicotine is highly poisonous and is sometimes used as an insecticide. Poisoning causes severe nausea and vomiting, spontaneous emptying of the bladder and bowels, mental confusion and convulsions. Nicotine does not cause cancer.

Like many other poisons, nicotine, taken in very small dosage, is valued for its stimulant properties. In smoking, the drug passes rapidly into the bloodstream and gives a quick 'lift' by its action on the brain until broken down in the liver and excreted in the urine. In people who are addicted, it increases the heart rate and raises the blood pressure by narrowing small arteries. This effect can be dangerous in certain arterial diseases.

Nicotine is not a powerfully addictive drug and those deprived of it have only minor withdrawal effects, which soon pass. Its use, nevertheless, is so important to many that they continue to smoke cigarettes although well aware of the appalling risk to health from the many other dangerous substances present in cigarette smoke.

Marijuana

This drug is obtained from various species of the hemp grass cannabis, especially *Cannabis sativa*. It is widely used and is generally believed to be harmless. Its main effect is to produce euphoria – easy laughter or giggling, often for reasons that seem silly or childish to the observer. There is an apparent heightening of all the senses, especially vision. Colour intensity and contrast are increased, and there is distortion of the dimensions of objects and of the perception of distance. The perception of time, too, is distorted, or sometimes seemingly eliminated. Usually, time seems to pass more slowly than normal.

One of the much-valued properties among the seekers for truth is the sense of philosophical insight conveyed by cannabis. The effect is, of course, an illusion. In fact, intellectual performance is impaired during the period of the drug action. Mental arithmetic is less accurate than normal and short-term memory weakened. The affected person often forgets the beginning of a sentence before reaching the end.

Cannabis has some important dangers. It causes widening of blood vessels, a fall in blood pressure and an increase in the heart rate. The effects on the heart can be dangerous and people with heart disease have suffered angina pectoris, heart failure and even death. In those not accustomed to it, cannabis can produce panic attacks or acute anxiety and it has often precipitated a state of depersonalization, true schizophrenia, mania, or a severe confusional psychosis. In most cases, these effects occur in people who might have developed the disorders, in due course, without cannabis. But sometimes they occur in those with no apparent psychiatric problem. Young teenagers, especially those under social or other stresses and those suffering emotional disturbances are especially at risk. Psychiatric patients controlled on drug treatment often suffer recurrences on using cannabis.

Reefer smoke can cause lung cancer and chronic bronchitis. In animals it causes damage to chromosomes, impairs cell division and causes abnormalities in the growing fetus, in doses equivalent to those commonly used in man. Happily, there have, so far, been no signs of genetic defects or fetal abnormalities in humans. But there is good evidence that cannabis increases the likelihood of early spontaneous abortion. The effect of medicinal drugs may be prolonged by cannabis, sometimes dangerously.

The question of organic brain damage remains controversial. This does occur in rats and monkeys, but has not been proved in humans. There is however, plenty of evidence of a damaging effect on brain function in persistent heavy users. Such people often show apathy and loss of interest and concern. Students stop working, suffer a drop in academic performance and give up courses (the amotivational syndrome). Cannabis withdrawal produces quite severe symptoms. These include:

- anxiety
- irritability
- headaches
- sleeplessness
- muscle twitching
- sweating
- diarrhoea

These symptoms will, however, pass and, in most cases, motivation eventually returns. The effect on performance is important. Slowing of reflexes, distortion of distance and alteration in the sense of responsibility all have a serious effect on skilled activities such as driving, patient monitoring, air traffic controlling, military surveillance, and so on. It is right that the public should be protected against the use of cannabis by people engaged in these activities. There is little evidence that cannabis promotes criminal activity.

Only a small proportion of casual cannabis users progress to harder drugs, but heavy users commonly do progress. Nearly all heroin addicts have had previous experience of cannabis, and the cannabis experience, in certain predisposed individuals, does cause progression, for psychological reasons, to drugs such as heroin.

Crack

Crack is a highly purified and powerful form of cocaine which is volatile on heating and is readily absorbed through the lungs. It acts like amphetamine, causing a 'high' with a short period of intense pleasure. This feeling is strongest on the first use and is never experienced to the same intensity again.

The use of crack quickly leads to dependence in some users and there is no way of knowing, in advance, who will become addicted and who will not. Some people seem to have little difficulty in keeping usage under control, but around 15 per cent of users just go on taking larger and larger doses until they are as dependent on the drug as heroin addicts.

The likelihood of severe addiction depends on the way the drug is used. People who are 'freebasing' (smoking) or 'shooting' (injecting) are much more likely to become seriously addicted than those who are only 'snorting' the drug. The trouble is that habituation and tolerance to the effect may lead snorters to want the extra 'rush' of freebasing, in which 80% of the dose can get to the brain in about 10 seconds. As with any other major drug of addiction, quite apart from its medical effects, habituation may lead to serious social and financial consequences. It is hardly necessary to mention the fact that an enormous amount of crime is directly attributable to the drug culture.

Many people choose to believe that crack is harmless, but it is, in fact, often dangerous to health. The commonest serious physical effects are:

- epileptic-type fits
- loss of consciousness ('tripping out')
- unsteadiness
- sore throat
- running and bleeding nose
- perforation of the nasal septum
- sinusitis
- pain in the chest
- coughing blood
- pneumonia

- severe itching ('the cocaine bug')
- irregularity of the heart
- loss of appetite
- stomach upset

Some of the chest and throat problems are probably caused by the high temperature of the inhaled cocaine fumes. The nose and sinus disorders are due to the constricting effect of cocaine on the blood vessels in the nose linings.

Crack, like amphetamine, can lead to a short-lived, acute form of mental illness. This is called a cocaine psychosis. The symptoms include severe depression, agitation, delusions, ideas of persecution, hallucinations, violent behaviour and suicidal intent. People with a cocaine psychosis often have 'lucid intervals' in which they seem normal and will often deny using the drug. Cocaine psychosis usually follows long binges or high doses.

Heroin

This drug is a chemically modified form of morphine. When first taken it causes nausea, vomiting and anxiety, but people who really try soon find that the drug gives them a euphoric 'high'. Tolerance soon develops so that more and more of the drug is needed to achieve the 'high'. So people who start by smoking the drug soon have to resort to injections under the skin and then to injections directly into the bloodstream. By this stage the withdrawal symptoms, experienced when the drug is not taken, are getting to be fairly severe. They include:

- restlessness
- anxiety
- irritability
- depression
- yawning
- sweating
- watering eyes
- nausea and vomiting

- cramping pains in the tummy
- diarrhoea
- aching bones
- shaking
- cold sweats with goose flesh ('cold turkey')
- insomnia
- sometimes seizures and collapse

Soon the chief concern is to avoid these withdrawal effects, and the addict's primary concern in life is to keep up a regular supply of the drug at all costs. The risks inherent in the repeated casual use of intravenous drugs, often by means of shared needles, need hardly be mentioned. Many heroin addicts kick the habit only to die later of AIDS. If a heroin addict stops completely and avoids methadone the withdrawal symptoms all settle in about 10 days.

Psychedelic drugs

'Acid' is lysergic acid diethylamide (LSD), a derivative of ergot. Other psychedelic drugs include mescaline, psilocybin, dimethyl- and diethyl-tryptamine, harmine, phencyclidine (PCP or 'angel dust') and various 'designer drugs' derived from amphetamine. Only very tiny doses of these drugs are needed and these produce mental effects within one or two hours. The effects vary with the state of mind of the user and with the surroundings, and include:

- distortion of time and space
- heightened perceptions of colours
- abnormal sharpness of images
- confusion of sounds and colours
- sense of bodily distortion
- sense of increased awareness
- illusory feelings of the high significance of ordinary matters

The effect on mood may vary from euphoria to depression or panic. Occasionally, very severe panic attacks occur ('bad trips') and these sometimes lead to suicide. People using these drugs quickly develop tolerance, but addiction is uncommon. Those who do become dependent sometimes develop a persistent psychiatric disorder (psychosis). The psychedelic drugs are liable to cause a strange phenomenon – a brief period of the return of the psychedelic effect, without warning and without having taken the drug. This is known as 'flashback'.

The major risks with phencyclidine are from abnormal behaviour – aggression, violence, reckless driving and so on. People affected by the drug may suffer serious falls or burns or die from drowning.

Benzodiazepines

If you take any benzodiazepine drug, such as diazepam (Valium), chlordiazepoxide (Librium), medazepam (Nobrium), chlorazepate (Tranxene), temazepam (Normison) or nitrazepam (Mogadon), for more than about six weeks, you are likely to become dependent. Withdrawal of the drug will then probably cause you quite severe symptoms. If you have become heavily dependent, withdrawal will probably cause:

- shakiness
- nausea
- headache
- sweating
- a sense of unreality
- excessive sensitivity to noise or bright light
- anxiety
- insomnia

These symptoms usually last for about two weeks, but sometimes go on for months. If you have become addicted to one of the benzodiazepines, you are going to need to have the drug withdrawn very gradually.

6. MISCELLANEOUS INFORMATION

Doctors have always been inclined to make a mystique of prescriptions but there is no good reason for this. You are entitled to know, and indeed *ought* to know, what you are being given and what it is likely to do to you.

Understanding prescriptions

A prescription is nothing more than a note from a doctor to a dispensing chemist (pharmacist), telling him or her what to do. There was a time, not so very long ago, when prescriptions were written in Latin so that ignorant people would not be able to understand them. Most pharmacists would have a problem with any doctor who did that nowadays. But some prescriptions still start with an odd symbol consisting of a capital R with a stroke across the tail of the letter. This was an abbreviation of the Latin *recipe* meaning 'take thou' and was originally followed by a string of ingredients that the apothecary was to use to concoct the medicine. Very few, if any, pharmaceutical chemists now make up medicines in this way. So the prescription of today tends to be quite a lot shorter and easier to deal with than that of the past.

Prescriptions are, however, important and, however quickly scribbled, are made with care. They must contain:

- your name and address
- the date of writing
- a precise statement of the drug to be dispensed
- the form the drug is to take (tablets, capsules, injection, drops, suppositories, ointments, etc.)
- the weight of drug in each tablet or capsule, or the total weight of ointment, etc, to be dispensed
- a statement of how much you are to take and how often
- any special instructions about how the drug should be taken
- the doctor's signature
- the doctor's name and address

Another hangover of the days of Latin prescriptions is the use of a range of abbreviations, many of which were originally in Latin and so are doubly mysterious. Here are a few abbreviations commonly used in prescriptions:

a.c. (ante cibum) before food
p.c. (post cibum) after food
o.d. (omni die) once a day
b.i.d. (bis in die) twice a day
t.i.d. (ter in die) three times a day
t.d.s. (ter die summendum) three times a day
q.i.d. (quater in die) four times a day
q.d.s. (quater die summendum) four times a day
mane in the morning
o.m. (omni mane) every morning
nocte at night
o.n. (omni nocte) every night
stat. (statim) immediately
p.o. (per os) by mouth
p.r. (per rectum) to be inserted through the anus
p.v. (per vaginam) to be inserted into the vagina
p.r.n. (pro re nata) as required
c (cum) with
s (sine) without
ad lib (ad libitum) take as much as you like
gutt. (guttae) drops
tab. tablet
caps. capsule
mist. (mistura) a mixture
ung (unguentum) an ointment
crem (cremor) a cream
oc (oculentum) an eye ointment

Whether these are helpful or not will depend on whether you are able to read your doctor's handwriting. Fortunately, pharmacists get to be very good at this. If they are in any doubt, however, they will always ring up the doctor concerned. It isn't really necessary for you to be able to read the doctor's prescription as the full instructions will be printed on the label of the medication by the pharmacist's computer.

How to store and safeguard drugs

When you have a prescription made up, check to see that the expiry date on the medication is well ahead. Drugs do not suddenly lose all their potency on the expiry date, but after that date, you can't be sure that they are satisfactory. If the date has passed, or if it is likely to do so before you have finished the course, point this out to the chemist and you will get a newer sample. If drugs show any sign of deterioration, ask for a fresh supply.

If possible, always keep drugs in the containers in which they were dispensed, so that the labels will apply to the contents. If you have to put them in something else, keep the original container. Always close up bottles and jars tightly. Many drugs will deteriorate more rapidly in an open container. If there is a silica gel desiccant in the container, leave it in place. Some of these desiccants look like large tablets, so be careful not to swallow one by mistake. It will not kill you, if you do.

The higher the temperature, the more rapidly most drugs will deteriorate. So find a reasonably cool place to keep your medicines, preferably out of the light and certainly out of reach of children. A high, lockable wall cabinet is ideal. Steamy bathrooms are not the best place for drugs. If you can spare a corner of the refrigerator your medicines will keep in perfect condition. A few drugs *must* be kept in the fridge.

Don't keep old drugs after you have finished with them. Flush them down the toilet. The dustbin is *not* the place for drugs of any kind. Get rid of any drugs that appear to have changed in any way, especially if they have developed a new smell. Capsules that have become sticky and softened should be disposed of. Eyedrops are not easy to sterilize and are easily contaminated. As a rule, they should be discarded a month after the bottle is first opened.

Remember that most suicides are achieved with drugs. You should bear this possibility in mind if anyone in your family is severely depressed. Watch out for obvious accumulation of drugs, especially sedatives. If young people are involved, lock away all drugs. Paracetamol is especially dangerous (see p. 40).

Poisoning with drugs

The first thing to do is to call an ambulance so as to get the victim to hospital as soon as possible, together with all available evidence of the type of poisoning – empty bottles, syringes, samples of vomit, tablets, etc. Inform the ambulance people that it is a poisoning case and state whether or not the victim is conscious. If you decide to take the victim by car, get someone to telephone the hospital casualty department or emergency room and warn them.

If you are delayed you can get urgent advice from a poison centre. It is important to know what the victim has taken before you call. It is natural to panic but you can save a lot of grief by taking a few deep breaths and trying to keep as calm as possible.

There are poison centres in major cities. Here is a current list for UK and Republic of Ireland:

Belfast: Royal Victoria Hospital, Grosvenor Road BT12 6BA. (0232) 240503 ext. 2140
Birmingham: West Midlands Poisons Unit, Dudley Road Hospital B18 7QH. (021) 554 3801 ext 4109
Cardiff: Welsh National Poisons Unit, Llandough Hospital, Penarth. (0222) 709901
Dublin: Poisons Information Centre, Beaumont Hospital, Beaumont Road. (0103531) 379966
Edinburgh: Edinburgh Royal Infirmary, EH3 9YW. (031) 2477 ext. 4786
Leeds: Poisons Information Service, General Infirmary, Great George Street LS1 3EX. (0532) 430715 or (0532) 432799 ext. 3547
London: New Cross Hospital, Avonley Road, SE14 5ER. (071) 635 9191
Newcastle: Royal Victoria Infirmary, NE1 4LP. (091) 232 1525 (day) or (091) 232 5131 (night)

If abroad, get someone who speaks the language well to telephone the nearest hospital emergency room for advice. If possible, get the poisoned person to hospital with the minimum of delay.

Drug overdose usually occurs in an attempt at suicide, but occasionally is the result of misinterpretation of medical instructions or, rarely, because of a mistake in prescription or dispensing. Certain drugs are taken in overdose more often than others. These, with the general symptoms and signs, include the following.

Amphetamines (Benzedrine, Dexedrine) – jumpiness, excitement, confusion, aggression, hallucinations.

Barbiturates (Amytal, Luminal, Seconal) – drowsiness, coma, hypothermia, slow and shallow breathing.

Benzodiazepines (Valium, Librium) – staggering, dizziness, drowsiness, shallow breathing.

Beta blockers (Sectral, Visken, Angilol) – very slow pulse, collapse, drowsiness, delirium, seizures, cardiac arrest.

Cocaine (Crack) – excitement, euphoria, restlessness, feelings of power, tremor, wide pupils, fast pulse, overbreathing, cardiac arrest.

Cyanide – smell of bitter almonds, shallow breathing, pink skin, wide pupils, shock, cardiac arrest.

Digoxin (Lanoxin) – nausea, vomiting, diarrhoea, yellow vision, slow irregular pulse.

Iron (Ferrocap, Ferromyn) – abdominal pain, nausea, vomiting, rapid pulse, black stools.

Lithium (Camcolit, Priadel) – nausea, vomiting, apathy, tremor, muscle twitching, convulsions.

NSAIDs (Brufen, Ebufac) – nausea, vomiting, abdominal pain, headache, rapid breathing, disorientation, jerking eyes, seizures, drowsiness, coma, cardiac arrest.

Paracetamol (Panadol) – nausea and vomiting. After 36 hours, acute liver failure may occur which is often fatal.

Salicylates (Aspirin) – deafness, ringing in the ears, blurring of vision, profuse sweating, cardiac arrest. Coma in children.

Tricyclic antidepressants (Tofranil, Tryptizol) – dry mouth, wide pupils, inability to urinate, hallucinations, twitching, loss of consciousness.

In most cases of recent drug poisoning it is helpful to make the victim vomit so as to try to get rid of as much of the poison as possible. This will be the case with most drug poisonings. Never induce vomiting if the poisoning is due to a corrosive poison such as strong acids or alkalis. In these cases, vomiting increases the risk of perforation of the stomach and additional damage to the gullet. In such a case, get the victim to drink four glasses of milk or water as soon as possible. Don't try to neutralize corrosives.

Never induce vomiting if poisoning is due to volatile substances like white spirit, essential oils or petroleum products. In these cases, vomiting encourages breathing in of the poison. You should never induce vomiting if the victim is in coma or could in any way inhale the vomit. If you decide to make someone vomit, be sure that he or she is leaning well forward.

You can usually induce vomiting by firmly stroking the back of the throat with a finger, as far down as you can. Don't use salty water. The most useful and effective household vomiting agent, however, is ipecacuanha. Paediatric syrup of ipecac, (not ipecac fluid extract which is 14 times as strong and is dangerous), should be used. This is available, without prescription, in 15 ml and 30 ml quantities. Children up to age 12 years need 15 ml. Older children and adults need 30 ml. The dose should be followed by a large drink of water. Ipecac takes 15 to 30 minutes to work. It contains the drug emetine which can affect the heart, but the risk is minor and is much less than the risk from a large overdose of drugs.

You should be constantly checking that the victim is conscious and breathing. If unconscious but breathing, the victim must be put into the 'recovery position'. This position prevents disastrous inhalation of vomit. Put the victim face down, head turned to one side and with one leg drawn up with the knee bent to prevent rolling over.

If breathing stops, you must turn the victim over onto his or her back and perform mouth-to-mouth resuscitation. Squeeze the nose, seal around the mouth with your mouth and blow up the lungs with one big blow. You must watch the chest rising to ensure that you are doing it properly. Let the lungs collapse and empty normally, then repeat at the rate of about 12 blows per minute. Check the victim's pulse with your fingertips down the side of the Adam's apple in the neck.

If you are absolutely sure that there is no pulse you will have to try to maintain the circulation and re-start the heart by external heart compression. Don't try this if the heart is beating very feebly, as external compression could stop the heart. The victim must be flat on his or her back. Put one hand centrally just above the angle of the ribs and your other hand on top of the first. Don't bend your elbows. Lean on the chest so that it goes in about 1 to 2 inches. This will squeeze the heart between the breast-bone and the spine and will push the blood round the circulation. You have to do this about 80 times a minute and give two mouth-to-mouth blows after every 15 chest compressions. This is very hard work. Get help with it if you can. If you have help, get the chest inflated after every 5 compressions. Timing is essential. Don't try to blow in while the chest is being compressed.

Drugs that can harm a fetus

About 3% of cases of congenital abnormality are believed to be due to drugs taken by the mother in early pregnancy. No drug can be considered entirely safe in pregnancy. The early fetus is highly sensitive to many drugs. Doctors are rightly very cautious about prescribing in pregnancy. Happily, no other drug has been found to cause such devastating or such frequent effects as thalidomide (see Chapter 1).

The following drugs are known to be capable of causing birth defects or of harming the fetus in other ways:

- Aspirin and NSAIDs (see below)
- alcohol
- heroin

- cocaine
- mumps, measles, rubella and polio vaccines
- oral contraceptives
- lithium
- isotretinoin
- diethylstilboestrol
- methotrexate
- disulfiram (Antabuse)
- danazole
- warfarin
- phenytoin
- sodium valproate
- vitamin A in high dosage
- sex hormones
- streptomycin
- barbiturates
- carbamazepine
- meprobamate
- certain cough medications

This list is far from complete. Every drug should be suspected and avoided if possible, especially in early pregnancy. There are risks in late pregnancy too. Aspirin and the NSAIDs (see Chapter 2) should never be taken in the last three months of pregnancy as they are liable to prolong labour and cause excessive bleeding during delivery. They are not thought to cause abnormalities in the fetus.

Breast feeding

Most drugs appear in the breast milk and several drugs can harm a baby if taken by a breast-feeding mother. These include:

- lithium
- chloromycetin
- tetracycline antibiotics
- sulphonamides
- anticancer drugs

- barbiturates
- iodides
- vitamins A or D in high dosage
- Aspirin in high dosage
- meprobamate
- sedatives
- ergot preparations

Again, the list is not exhaustive. Try to avoid drugs if you are breast feeding. Incidentally, urine-promoting (diuretic) drugs, sex hormones and bromocriptine (see Chapter 7) may stop the milk.

7. THE A TO Z GLOSSARY OF DRUGS AND THEIR ACTIONS

It would be a real enthusiast who would actually read right through this chapter, but no book of this kind could pretend to be much use if it did not contain the information included here. Some of the drugs listed are very recent and are still being evaluated, but all have been licensed for use.

Some drug names are printed with a capital initial letter, some with a lower case. This is a medical convention used to distinguish trade names (capital letter) from official or generic drug names (lower case). A generic drug is the 'official', approved, non-proprietary, and usually cheaper form of a single substance. The generic name is nearly always different from the name under which the drug is marketed (the trade or brand name), and there is often a range of different proprietary names – and prices – for the identical generic drug. Different manufacturers sell the same drug under different names.

Thus, 'paracetamol' is the generic name of the common painkilling (analgesic) drug Panadol, also known as Calpol, Pamol, Panasorb and Salzone. To make matters worse, the generic name of a drug is seldom a true chemical name. Acetaminophen, which is also paracetamol, sounds like a chemical name, but the real chemical name of paracetamol is 4'-hydroxyacetanilide.

Many proprietary preparations contain mixtures or combinations of generic drugs. Paracetamol is one of the main agents in Cafadol, Carisoma Co, Cosalgesic, Delimon, Distalgesic, Femerital, Fortagesic, Lobak, Medocodene, Myolgin, Neurodyne, Norgesic, Paedo-sed, Paracodol, Panadeine, Parahypon, Parake, Paralgin, Paramol-118, Para-selzer, Parazolidin, Pardale, Paxidal, Pharmidone, Propain, Safapryn, Solpadeine, Syndol, Tandalgesic, Unigesic, Veganin and Zactipar. This is a list, by no means exhaustive, of combinations of paracetamol with such other drugs as Aspirin, caffeine, codeine and phenylbutazone. The international drug directory *Index Nominum* lists 220 different names for paracetamol and 300 for Aspirin.

Official publications, such as the *British National Formulary*, express disapproval of these compound preparations, as they tend unnecessarily to increase the cost of treatment and may make it more difficult for doctors dealing with cases of overdosage. All drugs of medical value are available in the generic form and some doctors prescribe generic drugs only. But the overwhelming advertising pressures to which doctors are constantly exposed make such saintly behaviour as rare as it is difficult.

The drug names you are most likely to come across as a consumer, therefore, are the brand names under which drugs are commonly dispensed or bought. A great many of the commonest brand names are included in the following list. Unfortunately, the number of these names and of the names of combinations of drugs is so great that no book of this kind can include them all. If you look up a drug under a trade name you may be annoyed to find that you are immediately referred to the official name. There is really no practical way round this. There are several, sometimes dozens or scores, of trade names for every generic name. It would not be practicable to repeat the description of the drug for each one.

If the trade name you have in mind is not listed, don't worry. There is another way round the problem. By law, every prescription drug carries, somewhere on its packaging or container, a note of its generic name. You can find this after the words 'Active ingredients:' or perhaps after 'Contains . . .' or there may be a statement such as 'Each tablet contains . . . '. Often the generic name simply appears on its own. It is always a good idea to check to find out the real name of the drug you are taking. Then you will be in no doubt and can read all about it in this book.

Although the great majority of the drugs listed here can be obtained only on prescription there are a few non-prescription drugs that are so important that they have had to be included. There is a growing tendency, at present, to increase the number of formerly prescription-only drugs that can be bought over the counter. These drugs that are being released from restriction are carefully selected for their safety, but you should remember that no drug is safe if taken in more than the recommended dosage.

With so many drugs to cover, there is room for only a short description here. Don't forget to turn to Chapter 3, however, where you will probably find all you need to know about the action of a drug by looking under the appropriate drug group. You might also be interested to get an idea of how the drug you are concerned with actually brings about its effect on your body. You will find this information, too, in Chapter 3. Words in small capital letters are cross references to entries in this chapter.

Abbocillin – a trade name for PHENOXYMETHYLPENICILLIN.

Accubron – a trade name for THEOPHYLLINE.

acarbose – a glucosidase inhibitor drug used to treat maturity onset (Type II) diabetes that is inadequately controlled by diet or by other drugs. It is taken by mouth. Possible side effects include digestive upsets, a feeling of fullness, abdominal pain and diarrhoea. A trade name is Glucobay.

Accutane – a trade name for the anti-acne vitamin A-type drug ISOTRETINOIN. This drug can cause fetal abnormalities.

acebutolol – a beta-blocker drug commonly used to treat high blood pressure, angina pectoris and irregularity of the heart. It is taken by mouth. Possible side effects include breathing difficulty, especially in asthmatics, and cold hands and feet. A trade name is Sectral.

acecainide – a drug used to control irregularity of the heart.

acedapsone – a drug used to treat leprosy.

acemetacin – a drug used to treat rheumatoid arthritis and osteoarthritis. It is taken by mouth. Possible side effects include headaches, dizziness, chest pain, digestive upsets and ringing in the ears. A trade name is Emflex.

Acepril – a trade name for CAPTOPRIL.

acetaminophen – see PARACETAMOL.

acetazolamide – a urine-promoting (diuretic) drug that is, however, used almost exclusively in the treatment of glaucoma when the pressure rise inside the eyes cannot be controlled with eyedrops alone. The drug is also sometimes used in the treatment of epilepsy and periodic paralysis. A trade name is Diamox.

acetohexamide – a drug used to treat diabetes that does not require insulin, i.e. Type II (maturity-onset) diabetes. A trade name is Dymelor.

acetophenazine – an antipsychotic drug.

Acetopt – eye drops containing the sulpha drug SULPHACETAMIDE.

acetylcysteine – a drug used to reduce the thickness and stickiness of mucus. It is useful for freeing sputum in bronchitis and in liquefying mucus in cystic fibrosis. It is also used to improve eye comfort in some kinds of conjunctivitis. A trade name is Mucomyst.

acetylsalicylic acid – the common painkilling drug Aspirin. It also has valuable properties in reducing the stickiness of blood platelets, thus lowering the risk of clotting within the blood vessels. This can prevent coronary thrombosis, but may increase the chances of stroke. Aspirin is an antiprostaglandin drug and has anti-inflammatory as well as painkilling properties. In addition, it can reduce fever. New uses for Aspirin are regularly found. It is taken by mouth. Possible side effects include digestive upsets, bleeding from the stomach lining, Reye's syndrome (a serious brain and liver disorder) in children, promotion of bleeding and prolongation of labour in childbirth, and allergies.

Achromycin – a trade name for TETRACYCLINE.

Achrostatin – a trade name for TETRACYCLINE and NYSTATIN.

acipimox – a vitamin B derivative used to treat high blood cholesterol. It is taken by mouth. Possible side effects include skin rash, flushing, headache and sickness. A trade name is Olbetam.

acitretin – another name for ACLARUBICIN.

aclarubicin – an antimitotic (anticancer) drug administered by injection. Possible side effects include nausea and vomiting, loss of hair and interference with bone marrow blood cell production. A trade name is Aclacin.

Acnacyl – a trade name for BENZOYL PEROXIDE.

Acnegel – a trade name for BENZOYL PEROXIDE.

acriflavine – an orange powder derived from acridine and used, in solution, as an antiseptic for skin cleansing and wound washing.

acrivastine – an antihistamine drug used to treat hay fever and urticaria. It is taken by mouth. Possible side effects include drowsiness. A trade name is Semprex.

acrosoxacin – an antibiotic drug used to treat gonorrhoea. It is taken by mouth. Possible side effects include drowsiness, headache, dizziness and digestive upset. A trade name is Eradacin.

Actacode – a trade name for CODEINE.

Actifed – a trade name for a combination of TRIPROLIDINE and PSEUDOEPHEDRINE.

Actilyse – the tissue plasminogen activator drug ALTEPLASE.

actinomycin D – a toxic antibiotic used to treat cancer. Possible side effects include nausea, vomiting, hair loss and interference with blood cell production. A trade name is Cosmegen Lyovac.

activated charcoal – a highly absorbent form of carbon used to absorb gas, to deodorize and to inactivate various poisons that have been swallowed.

Actraphane – a trade name for a form of INSULIN.

Actrapid – a trade name for a form of INSULIN.

Actuss – a trade name for PHOLCODEINE.

Acupan – a trade name for NEFOPAM.

acyclovir – a drug that attacks the *Herpes simplex* virus and the closely similar chickenpox and shingles virus (the varicella-zoster virus). Early treatment with the drug, taken by mouth, can greatly reduce the severity of shingles and minimize the pain felt afterwards. A trade name is Zovirax.

Adalat – a trade name for NIFEDIPINE.

adrenaline – an important natural body hormone that is used as a sympathomimetic drug. It has many uses, including the treatment of acute allergic reactions and of the severe narrowing of the air tubes in asthma. It is also used to tighten small blood vessels so as to prevent the absorption of local anaesthetics, to strengthen the action of the heart and to treat certain forms of raised pressure within the eyes (glaucoma). Also known as epinephrine. Trade names are Eppy, Medihaler-Epi, Simplene.

Aerocrom – a trade name for a compound of CROMOGLYCATE and SALBUTAMOL.

agar – a seaweed derivative used to treat constipation. It is taken by mouth. Possible side effects include allergic reactions, blood cell damage. A trade name is Agarol.

albendazole – an anthelmintic drug used to get rid of roundworms, hookworms and other worm parasites. It is taken by mouth. Possible side effects include headache, dizziness, fever, skin rashes and loss of hair. A trade name is Eskazole.

albuterol – a drug that widens the air tubes and is used in the treatment of asthma, bronchitis and emphysema. A trade name is Ventolin.

alclometazone – a corticosteroid drug administered externally as a cream or ointment to treat inflammatory skin disorders. Possible side effects include skin thinning and allergic reactions. A trade name is Modrasone.

alcuronium – a neuromuscular blocking drug causing profound muscle relaxation. It is used by anaesthetists and administered by injection. Possible side effects include delay in resuming spontaneous breathing, so that artificial ventilation is needed. A trade name is Alloferin.

aldesleukin – human interleukin (interleukin 2) produced by recombinant DNA technology (genetic engineering). Interleukins act to enhance the function of the immune system. Aldesleukin prompts T lymphocytes to become cytotoxic (killer) cells, active against cancer cells. It is administered by injection. The results against certain cancers such as melanomas and kidney cell cancer have been encouraging. A trade name is Proleukin.

alfacalcidol – a synthetic form of vitamin D used to treat low blood calcium and osteomalacia caused by kidney disease. It is taken by mouth or given by injection. A trade name is One-alpha.

alfentanil hydrochloride – a narcotic analgesic drug used to relieve severe pain. It is administered by injection. A trade name is Rapifen.

alfuzocin – an alpha-blocker drug used to treat urinary difficulty from enlargement of the prostate gland. It is taken by mouth. Possible side effects include dizziness, headache, palpitations, chest pain, drowsiness and rashes. A trade name is Xatral.

alginic acid – an antacid drug used to treat heartburn caused by acid reflux into the gullet and hiatus hernia. It is taken by mouth. A trade name is Gastrocote, Gastron.

allantoin – a drug used externally, in combination with other substances, to treat psoriasis. Possible side effects include skin irritation. A trade name is Alphosyl.

allopurinol – a drug used to treat gout. Trade names are Zyloric, Lopurin, Zyloprim.

allyloestrenol – a progestogen drug used to treat threatened or habitual miscarriage or premature labour. It is taken by mouth. Possible side effects include nausea. A trade name is Gestanin.

aloin – a drug used to treat constipation. It is taken by mouth.

Possible side effects include allergic reactions and damage to red blood cells. A trade name is Alophen.

alprazolam – a long-acting benzodiazepine drug used to treat anxiety and depression. It is taken by mouth. Possible side effects include drowsiness, confusion, urinary retention, visual upset and loss of sexual interest. A trade name is Xanax.

alprostadil – a prostaglandin drug administered by injection to improve lung blood flow in newborn babies with congenital heart defects who are awaiting surgery. Possible side effects include diminished respiratory efforts. A trade name is Prostin VR.

alteplase – a tissue-type plasminogen activator drug made by recombinant DNA technology. The drug is used to dissolve blood clots in the circulation, especially in the coronary arteries of the heart. It is administered by injection. Possible side effects include local bleeding, cerebral haemorrhage, nausea and vomiting. A trade name is Actilyse.

aluminium acetate – a drug used externally to reduce perspiration. Trade names are Anhydrol Forte, Driclor.

aluminium dihydroxyallantoinate – a drug used externally as a dusting powder to treat excessive perspiration and skin damage from moisture and friction. A trade name is Zeasorb.

aluminium hydroxide – an antacid drug that reacts with stomach acid to form an insoluble compound, thereby reducing the amount of acid present. The drug tends to be constipating and may be dangerous if taken in excess especially in people with kidney disorders. A trade name is Aludrox.

aluminium oxide – a compound used externally as an abrasive cleansing paste to treat acne. A trade name is Brasivol.

alverine citrate – a bulking agent and antispasmodic drug used to treat irritable bowel syndrome and other colonic disorders. It is taken by mouth. Possible side effects include occasional mild distention of the bowel. A trade name is Alvercol, Spasmonal.

amantadine hydrochloride – a drug used to relieve the symptoms of Parkinsonism and as an antiviral agent. It is taken by mouth. Possible side effects include skin rashes and discoloration, oedema, digestive disturbances and visual upset. A trade name is Symmetrel.

amikacin – an aminoglycoside antibiotic drug. A trade name is Amikin.

amiloride – a urine-promoting (diuretic) drug. Trade names are Burinex A, Frumil, Lasoride and Moduretic.

aminobenzoic acid – a drug used to prevent the formation of fibrous tissue in the hardening skin disorder scleroderma and the penile distorting condition Peyronie's disease. It is taken by mouth. Possible side effects include nausea and loss of appetite. A trade name is Potaba.

aminoglutethimide – a drug that interferes with the body's production of steroids and is used to treat cancer. It is taken by mouth. Possible side effects include skin rashes, digestive upset, nervous system disorders and thyroid gland upset. A trade name is Orimeten.

aminophylline – a drug used to treat asthma and congestive heart failure. It is taken by mouth. Possible side effects include nausea, headache and digestive upset. Trade names are Pecram, Phyllocontin.

amiodarone – an anti-arrhythmic drug used to control a variety of abnormal heart rhythms such as fibrillation of the upper chambers (atrial fibrillation) or an abnormally rapid heartbeat. It is taken by mouth or given by injection. Side effects are uncommon. A trade name is Cordarone X.

amitriptyline – a tricyclic antidepressant drug. It is taken by mouth. Possible side effects include dry mouth, constipation, blurred vision and difficulty in urinating. Trade names are Domical, Elavil, Lentizol and Tryptizol.

amlodipine – a calcium antagonist drug used to treat angina pectoris. It is taken by mouth. Possible side effects include headache, dizziness, fatigue, nausea and fluid retention. A trade name is Istin.

amodiaquine – an antimalarial drug used in the event of quinine intolerance in CHLOROQUINE-resistant malaria.

amorolfine – an antifungal (antimycotic) drug administered as a cream for external use for the treatment of tinea, candidiasis and other skin fungal infections and for tinea of the nails. Possible side effects include itching and a transient burning sensation. A trade name is Loceryl.

amoxapine – a tricyclic antidepressant drug similar to imipramine. It is taken by mouth. Possible side effects include dry mouth, constipation, blurred vision and difficulty in urinating. Overdosage may cause acute kidney failure, convulsions and coma. A trade name is Asendis.

Amoxidin – a trade name for AMOXYCILLIN.

Amoxil – a trade name for AMOXYCILLIN.

amoxycillin – an AMPICILLIN-like penicillin antibiotic, effective in typhoid and many other infections. It is taken by mouth. Trade names are Amoxil, Larotid, Trimox, Utimox.

amphetamine – a central nervous system stimulant drug with few medical uses but commonly abused to obtain a 'high'. Amphetamine use leads to tolerance and sometimes physical dependence. Overdosage causes irritability, tremor, restlessness, insomnia, flushing, nausea and vomiting, irregularity of the pulse, delirium, hallucinations, convulsions and coma. Amphetamine can precipitate a psychosis in predisposed people.

Amphogel – a trade name for ALUMINIUM HYDROXIDE.

amphotericin-B – an antibiotic drug used to treat fungal infections within the body. It is moderately toxic and side effects are common. A trade name is Fungilin.

ampicillin – a widely used PENICILLIN antibiotic, effective by mouth and capable of killing many organisms. About one third of the dose is excreted unchanged in the urine. The drug precipitates a characteristic rash if given to people incubating glandular fever (infective mononucleosis). A trade name is Penbritin.

Ampicyn – a trade name for AMPICILLIN.

Amprace – a trade name for ENALAPRIL.

amsacrine – a cytotoxic anticancer drug administered by injection. Possible side effects include nausea, vomiting, hair loss and interference with bone marrow blood cell production. A trade name is Amsidine.

amygdalin – a glycoside found in the stones of bitter almonds, from which LAETRILE was isolated.

amylobarbitone – a barbiturate drug still used occasionally to treat insomnia. It is taken by mouth. Possible side effects include drowsiness, dizziness, confusion and allergic reactions. A trade name is Amytal.

Amytal – a trade name for amylobarbitone, a barbiturate hypnotic drug of medium duration of action.

Anafranil – a trade name for CLOMIPRAMINE.

Anamorph – a trade name for MORPHINE.

Anapolon – a trade name for OXYMETHOLONE.

Ancolan – a trade name for MECLOZINE.

Ancoloxin – a trade name for MECLOZINE.

Ancotil – a trade name for FLUCYTOSINE.

Andriol – a trade name for TESTOSTERONE.

Andrumin – a trade name for DIMENHYDRINATE.

Anethaine – a trade name for AMETHOCAINE.

anethol – a mixture of essential oils used to treat mild urinary infections and stones in the urinary tract. It is taken by mouth. A trade name is Rowatinex.

aneurin – vitamin B1, thiamin (or thiamine). This is plentiful in cereals and fresh vegetables, beans, peas, fruit, meat and milk, but there is very little in refined foods, fat, sugar or alcohol. Deficiency causes beri-beri in one to two months. Also known as thiamine.

Angilol – a trade name for PROPRANOLOL.

Anginine – a trade name for GLYCERYL TRINITRATE.

anistreplase – a drug consisting of a complex of the clot-dissolving substances streptokinase and plasminogen. It is used to dissolve blood clots in the circulation. It is administered by injection. Possible side effects include local bleeding, slowing of the heart, flushing, low blood pressure, fever, nausea, vomiting and allergic reactions. A trade name is Eminase.

Anpec – a trade name for VERAPAMIL.

Antabuse – disulfiram. A drug sometimes used to try to control alcoholism. If people taking the drug have a drink, they will suffer severe nausea, vomiting, sweating, breathlessness, headache and chest pain. Disulfiram interferes with the enzyme that breaks down acetaldehyde, a poisonous product of alcohol, so that this accumulates. Antabuse treatment is called aversion therapy and is not entirely safe. Some patients have died from the poisonous effects.

Antadine – a trade name for AMANTADINE.

antazoline – an ANTIHISTAMINE drug that also has weak local anaesthetic effects. It is used in the form of eyedrops to treat allergic conjunctivitis. Possible side effects include stinging, headache, drowsiness and blurred vision. A trade name is Antistin-Privine.

Antenex – a trade name for DIAZEPAM.

Antepar – a trade name for PIPERAZINE.

Anthel – a trade name for PYRANTEL.

Anthisan – a trade name for MEPYRAMINE.

Anthranol – a trade name for DITHRANOL.

antitetanus serum – a serum containing specific antibodies against tetanus. It is usually obtained from a horse which has been inoculated with tetanus organisms and has developed immunity to the disease. People who have had proper tetanus immunization with tetanus toxoid do not need antitetanus serum, which can produce dangerous allergic reactions.

antivenin – an antiserum containing antibodies to the venom of poisonous snakes, scorpions or spiders. Also known as antivenene.

antivenom – see ANTIVENIN.

Antraderm – a trade name for DITHRANOL.

aperient – a laxative or mild purgative.

apomorphine – a drug made from morphine and used to treat Parkinson's disease and to assist in coughing up sputum. In large doses it promotes severe vomiting. This can be useful in poisoning. It is administered by injection. A trade name is Britaject.

apraclonidine – a drug used as eyedrops to treat raised pressure in the eyes (glaucoma). A trade name is Iopidine.

Apresoline – a trade name for HYDRALAZINE.

Aprinox – a trade name for BENDROFLUAZIDE.

aprotinin – a drug that prevents the breakdown of blood clots and helps to control bleeding. An antifibrinolytic drug administered by injection. A trade name is Trasylol.

ara-C – cytarabine, an antileukaemic drug.

arachis oil – a drug used as ear drops to soften ear wax, as a skin emulsion to treat dry skin, and as an enema to soften hard faeces. Trade names are Cerumol, Hydromol, Fletcher's arachis oil.

arsphenamine – a compound of arsenic formerly used to treat syphilis. Treatment with arsenical drugs was called arsenotherapy.

Artane – a trade name for BENZHEXOL.

Arthrexin – a trade name for INDOMETHACIN.

Artracin – a trade name for INDOMETHACIN.

Ascabiol – a trade name for BENZYL BENZOATE.

Ascalix – a trade name for PIPERAZINE.

ascorbic acid – vitamin C. A white, crystalline substance found in citrus fruits, tomatoes, potatoes, and leafy green vegetables. Small doses are needed to prevent the bleeding disease of scurvy and large doses are useful in combating free radicals.

Asilone – a trade name for ALUMINIUM HYDROXIDE.

Asmaven – a trade name for SALBUTAMOL.

aspartame – an artificial sweetener derived from aspartic acid and phenylalanine.

Aspirin – a trade name for ACETYLSALICYLIC ACID.

Aspro – a trade name for ACETYLSALICYLIC ACID (Aspirin).

Asprodeine – a trade name for a compound of Aspirin and CODEINE.

astemizole – an antihistamine drug used to treat hay fever and allergic skin conditions. It is taken by mouth. Possible side effects include weight gain and, on very high dosage, heart irregularity. A trade name is Hismanal.

atacurium besylate – a neuromuscular blocking drug used by anaesthetists that causes profound muscle relaxation. It is administered by injection. A trade name is Tracrium.

Atarax – a trade name for HYDROXYZINE.

atenolol – a beta-blocker drug that acts mostly on the heart and has a long action. It slows the heart and corrects irregularities of rhythm. Possible side effects include sleep disturbance, tiredness, digestive upset, cold hands and feet, asthma and undue slowing of the heart. A trade name is Tenormin.

Atensine – a trade name for DIAZEPAM.

Ativan – a trade name for LORAZEPAM.

atovaquone – a drug with strong action against *Toxoplasma gondii*, the organism that causes toxoplasmosis. Atovaquone appears to be well tolerated and has been used in AIDS patients to treat toxoplasmosis of the brain. Scans show considerable improvement.

atracurium besolate – a muscle relaxant used by anaesthetists. It is administered by injection. A trade name is Tracrium.

Atromid-S – a trade name for CLOFIBRATE.

atropine sulphate – a bitter, poisonous alkaloid obtained from the plant *Atropa belladonna* ('deadly nightshade') and the seeds of the thorn apple. It is used to relax spasm in muscle in the intestines (colic) and other organs. It is also extensively used by eye specialists to widen the pupil of the eye in the treatment of internal eye inflammation and sometimes to make it easier to examine the inside of the eye. It is taken by mouth or in eye drops. Possible side effects dry mouth, redness of the skin, absence of sweating and fever. Trade names are Belladonna, Lomotil, Minims atropine.

auranofin – a gold preparation used to treat rheumatoid arthritis. It is taken by mouth. Side effects include nausea, abdominal pain, diarrhoea and mouth ulcers. A trade name is Ridaura.

Aureomycin – the antibiotic CHLORTETRACYCLINE.

Austramycin – a trade name for TETRACYCLINE.

Austrapen – a trade name for AMPICILLIN.

autumn crocus – a plant, *Colchicum autumnale*, from which the valuable gout remedy colchicine is derived.

Avil – a trade name for PHENIRAMINE.

Avloclor – a trade name for CHLOROQUINE.

Avomine – a trade name for PROMETHAZINE.

Azactam – a trade name for AZTREONAM.

Azamune – a trade name for AZATHIOPRINE.

azapropazone – a non-steroidal anti-inflammatory drug (NSAID) used to treat rheumatoid arthritis, osteoarthritis, ankylosing spondylitis and gout. It is taken by mouth. Possible side effects include sensitivity of skin to light, fluid retention, bleeding from the bowel and a form of pneumonia (alveolitis). A trade name is Rheumox.

azatadine – an antihistamine and serotonin antagonist drug use to treat hay fever, urticaria, itching and stings. It is taken by mouth. Possible side effects include drowsiness, headache, nausea and loss of appetite. A trade name is Optimine.

azathioprine – a drug used to suppress the immune system so as to avoid rejection of donor transplant organs or tissue. Immune suppression may have serious side effects such as the flare-up of latent infections and an increased risk of cancer, especially lymphomas, but azathioprine is safer than other immunosuppressive drugs. Also used to treat rheumatism. A trade name is Imuran.

azelaic acid – an antibacterial drug administered as a cream for external application in the treatment of acne. Possible side effects include local irritation and light sensitivity. A trade name is Skinoren.

azelastine – an antihistamine drug administered as a metered-dose nasal spray for the treatment of hay fever. Possible side effects include nasal irritation and disturbances of taste sensation. A trade name is Rhinolast.

Azide – a trade name for CHLOROTHIAZIDE.

azithromycin – an antibiotic drug used to treat respiratory, skin, soft tissue and other infections, especially those caused by the organism *Chlamydia trachomatis*. It is taken by mouth. Possible side effects include allergic reactions, nausea and vomiting. A trade name is Zithromax.

azlocillin – an antibiotic drug, administered by intravenous infusion, to treat infections especially those caused by the dangerous organism *Pseudomonas aeruginosa*. Possible side effects include allergic reactions, nausea and vomiting. A trade name is Securopen.

AZT – azidothymidine or zidovudine. A drug used in attempts to control AIDS. The drug is poisonous but does seem to be able to prolong life.

aztreonam – an antibiotic drug used to treat infections of the lungs, bones, skin and soft tissues with organisms of the Gram stain negative class (Gram-negative organisms). It is especially useful in lung infections in children with cystic fibrosis. It is administered by injection. Possible side effects include skin rashes, diarrhoea and vomiting. A trade name is Azactam.

bacampicillin – a semisynthetic penicillin antibiotic. It is similar to ampicillin but is absorbed better so more of it gets into the blood.

bacitracin – an antibiotic made from the germ *Bacillus subtilis*. It works by preventing germs from forming a normal outer coat and is highly effective against many organisms. Unfortunately, it is very likely to damage the kidneys and is limited to external use.

baclofen – a drug similar to the body's nerve stimulator GABA. Baclofen damps down nerve action in the spinal cord and relaxes muscle spasm. It is used to alleviate the effects of stroke, multiple sclerosis and other conditions. A trade name is Lioresal.

Bactrim – a trade name for CO-TRIMOXAZOLE.

BAL – British antilewisite, or DIMERCAPROL.

bambuterol a drug used to relieve air tube spasm in asthma. It is taken by mouth. Possible side effects include headaches, tremor, cramps and palpitations. A trade name is Bambec.

Baratol – a trade name for INDORAMIN.

Barbopent – a trade name for PENTOBARBITONE.

Becloforte – a trade name for BECLOMETHASONE.

beclomethasone – a corticosteroid drug used in the form of a nasal spray, inhaler or ointment to relieve the symptoms of hay fever and asthma. Possible side effects include nasal irritation, sore throat and cough. Trade names are Beconase, Becotide, Propaderm.

Beconase – a trade name for BECLOMETHASONE.

Becotide – a trade name for BECLOMETHASONE.

belladonna – a crude form of ATROPINE derived from the leaves and roots of the poisonous plant, *Atropa belladonna*. The name comes from the cosmetic use of the alkaloid to widen the pupils. 'Bella donna' is Italian for 'beautiful woman'.

bendrofluazide – a urine-promoting (diuretic) drug used to treat high blood pressure and heart failure. It is taken by mouth. Possible side effects include digestive upset, loss of appetite, blood cell damage, impotence and dizziness. Trade names are Aprinox, Centyl and Inderex.

Benemid – a trade name for PROBENECID.

Benoral – a trade name for BENORYLATE.

benorylate – a drug derived from Aspirin and PARACETAMOL which is less irritating to the stomach than Aspirin, but equally effective as a painkiller and non-steroidal anti-inflammatory drug. A trade name is Benoral.

Benoxyl – a trade name for BENZOYL PEROXIDE.

benperidol – a butyrophenone antipsychotic drug used mainly to treat deviant and antisocial sexual behaviour. It is taken by mouth. A trade name is Anquil.

benserazide – a drug given in conjunction with LEVODOPA to prevent its breakdown in the body. It is used to treat Parkinsonism following encephalitis (post-encephalitic Parkinsonism). Side effects include nausea, vomiting, loss of appetite, involuntary movements and faintness on standing up. A trade name is Madopar.

Benylin – a trade name for DIPHENHYDRAMINE with other ingredients.

Benzac – a trade name for BENZOYL PEROXIDE.

Benzagel – a trade name for BENZOYL PEROXIDE.

benzalkonium – an antiseptic used in solution for skin and wound cleansing and to sterilize eye drops and contact lens solutions. Allergic reactions can occur. A trade name is Drapolene.

benzathine penicillin – an early, long-acting penicillin that must be given by injection.

Benzedrine – a trade name for AMPHETAMINE.

benzhexol – a drug that blocks the action of the body's natural nerve stimulant acetylcholine. It is used to treat the symptoms of Parkinson's disease, such as tremor and muscle tension.

benzocaine – a tasteless white powder with powerful local anaesthetic properties. Often used in lozenges in combination with antiseptics. A trade name is Tyrozets.

benzoyl peroxide – a preparation used in the treatment of acne and other skin conditions. It acts by removing the surface layers of the epidermis and unblocking skin pores, and has an antiseptic effect on skin bacteria. It is administered as a cream, lotion or gel. Side effects include skin irritation and excessive peeling, even, occasionally, blistering. Trade names are Acetoxyl, Acnegel, Benoxyl.

benztropine – a nerve-dampening drug used to control the symptoms of Parkinson's disease.

benzydamine hydrochloride – a non-steroidal anti-inflammatory drug (NSAID) used to treat muscle pain. It is administered as a cream for external use. A trade name is Difflam.

benzyl benzoate – a drug used as an oily liquid lotion for the treatment of scabies.

benzylpenicillin – the original highly active penicillin. The drug is destroyed by the digestive system and so must be given by injection.

bephenium hydroxynaphthoate – an anthelmintic drug to get rid of hookworms and other nematodes. It is taken by mouth. Possible side effects include stomach irritation. A trade name is Alcopar.

Berkatens – a trade name for VERAPAMIL.

Berkmycen – a trade name for OXYTETRACYCLINE.

Berocca – a trade name for a mixture of B vitamins and vitamin C.

Berotec – a trade name for FENOTEROL.

Betadine – the trade name for povidone iodine, a mild antiseptic, which is used as a surgical scrub or as a lotion or ointment.

Betadren – a trade name for PINDOLOL.

betahistine – a drug with properties similar to the natural body substance histamine, that is used to treat Ménière's disease. It is taken by mouth. A common side effect is nausea. A trade name is Serc.

betaine hydrochloride – a drug used in a compound with a potassium salt to treat potassium deficiency. It is taken by mouth. A trade name is Kloref.

Betaloc – a trade name for METOPROLOL.

betamethasone – a STEROID drug used directly on the skin to treat eczema and psoriasis; by inhalation to treat asthma; by mouth for more severe allergic conditions; and by injection to reduce brain swelling in head injuries, tumour and infections. Trade names are Betnesol and Betnovate.

Betamin – a trade name for THIAMINE.

betaxolol – a beta-blocker drug used to treat high blood pressure and chronic simple (open angle) glaucoma. It is taken by mouth and as eye drops. Possible side effects include breathing difficulty, fatigue, cold extremities and sleep disturbances. A trade name is Kerlone, Betoptic.

bethanechol – a cholinergic drug that acts mainly on the bowel and bladder, stimulating these organs to empty. It is taken by mouth. Possible side effects include nausea, vomiting, abdominal cramps, sweating and blurred vision. A trade name is Myotonine.

Betim – a trade name for TIMOLOL.

Betnelan – a trade name for BETAMETHASONE.

Betnesol – a trade name for BETAMETHASONE.

Betnovate – a trade name for BETAMETHASONE.

bezafibrate – a cholesterol-lowering drug used to treat abnormally high blood cholesterol levels (hypercholesterolaemia) that fail to respond to changes in diet. It is taken by mouth. Possible side effects include skin rash, nausea, vomiting and muscle pain. A trade name is Bezalip.

Bezalip – bezafibrate, a drug used to lower blood cholesterol levels.

Bicillin – benzathine penicillin.

BiCNU – a trade name for CARMUSTINE.

Biltricide – a trade name for PRAZIQUANTEL.

Biocitrin – vitamin C.

Bioplex – a trade name for CARBENOXOLONE.

Biotime – a mixture of vitamins and minerals.

Biovital – a mixture of vitamins and minerals.

Biphasil – an oral contraceptive.

Biquinate – a trade name for QUININE.

Bismag – a mixture of baking soda (SODIUM BICARBONATE) and MAGNESIUM CARBONATE.

bismuth – a drug used, as the carbonate, to treat peptic ulcer, especially cases in which the organism *Helicobacter pylori* is a causal agent. It is taken by mouth. Bismuth is also used, as the oxide or subgallate, for external use as a soothing ointment. Trade names are (carbonate) APP, (oxide) Anusol.

Bisodol – a trade name for a mixture of baking soda (sodium bicarbonate), chalk (calcium carbonate) and magnesium carbonate.

bisoprolol – a beta-blocker drug used to treat angina pectoris. It is taken by mouth. Possible side effects include breathing difficulty, fatigue, cold extremities and sleep disturbances. Trade names are Emcor, Monocor.

bithionol – a bacteriostatic agent useful against many organisms. It was formerly incorporated in medicated soaps. It is also used to treat parasitic diseases such as paragonimiasis.

Blenoxane – a trade name for BLEOMYCIN.

bleomycin – a rather poisonous antibiotic that interferes with DNA copying in the body and is used as an anticancer drug, usually in combination with other drugs. It is used to treat Hodgkin's disease, other lymphomas and some skin cancers (squamous cell cancers). The side effects include scarring (fibrosis) of the lungs and drying and discoloration of the skin around joints.

Blocadren – a trade name for TIMOLOL.

borneol – an essential oil used, in conjunction with other essential oils, such as menthol, menthone and camphene, to disperse gallstones and kidney stones. It is taken by mouth. Trade names are Rowachol, Rowatinex.

botulinum toxin – the powerful nerve toxin produced by the bacterium *Clostridium botulinum* which has been found valuable, in minute dosage, for the treatment of various conditions of muscle overaction such as strabismus and blepharospasm. It is administered by injection. Possible side effects include prolonged local muscle paralysis. A trade name is Dysport.

bretylium tosylate – a drug used in emergency to try to reverse the rapidly fatal ventricular fibrillation, a form of cardiac arrest, that has failed to respond to attempts at electrical defibrillation. It is administered by intravenous injection. A trade name is Bretylate.

Brevital – a short-acting BARBITURATE drug, methohexital sodium, used to put patients off to sleep in general anaesthesia.

Bricanyl – a trade name for TERBUTALINE.

Brinaldix – a trade name for CLOPAMIDE.

British antilewisite (BAL) – see DIMERCAPROL.

Brocadopa – a trade name for LEVODOPA.

Brolene – an eye ointment containing DIBROMOPROPAMIDINE.

bromazepam – a long-acting benzodiazepam drug used in the short-term treatment of disabling anxiety. It is taken by mouth. A trade name is Lexotan.

bromocriptine – an ergot derivative drug with dopamine-like effects. It is used in the treatment of Parkinson's disease and to prevent lactation by inhibiting the secretion of the hormone prolactin by the pituitary gland. The drug is taken by mouth. Fairly common side effects are dizziness and confusion. A trade name is Parlodel.

Brompton cocktail – a mixture of alcohol, morphine and cocaine sometimes given to control severe pain in terminally ill people, especially those dying of cancer. The mixture was first tried at the Brompton Hospital, London and has given relief to thousands.

bromsulphthalein – a substance used in a liver function test. The rate of clearance of bromsulphthalein from the blood, after injection, is a measure of liver efficiency. The test is now largely replaced by enzyme tests.

Brufen – a trade name for IBUPROFEN.

Brulidine – a preparation containing DIBROMOPROPAMIDINE.

budesonide – a corticosteroid drug used in a nasal spray for hay fever (allergic rhinitis) or as an inhalant for asthma. It is also administered as a cream or ointment for the treatment of eczema, psoriasis and other kinds of dermatitis. Trade names are Pulmicort (inhalant), Preferid (cream).

bufexamac – a non-steroidal anti-inflammatory drug (NSAID) administered externally in the form of a cream for the treatment of skin inflammation and to relieve itching. A trade name is Parfenac.

bumetanide – a quick-acting diuretic drug used to relieve the fluid retention (oedema) occurring in heart failure, kidney disease such as the nephrotic syndrome and cirrhosis of the liver. It is taken by mouth or given by injection. A possible side effect is dizziness. A trade name is Burinex.

bupivacaine – a long-acting local anaesthetic drug often used for nerve blocks, especially in epidural anaesthesia during childbirth and for the control of postoperative pain. A trade name is Marcaine.

buprenorphine – a powerful synthetic opiate painkilling drug that binds to the body's opioid receptors. It acts for 6–8 hours and is taken by mouth. Side effects include drowsiness, nausea, dizziness and sweating. A trade name is Temgesic.

buproprion – an antidepressant drug. A trade name is Wellbutrin.

Burinex – a trade name for BUMETANIDE.

Buscopan – a trade name for HYOSCINE.

buselerin – a drug that simulates the action of the gonadotrophin releasing hormone gonadorelin. It is administered as a nasal spray for the treatment of endometriosis and to help in the management of advanced cancer of the prostate gland. Possible side effects include hot flushes, vaginal dryness, headache, breast tenderness, emotional upset and loss of sexual interest. A trade name is Suprecur (women), Suprefact (men).

Buspar – a trade name for BUSPIRONE.

buspirone – a non-benzodiazepine antianxiety drug with slow onset of effect. A trade name is Buspar.

busulphan – an anticancer drug used especially in the treatment of chronic granulocytic leukaemia. It is poisonous and can destroy the function of the bone marrow unless its use is carefully monitored. It can also cause widespread scarring (fibrosis) of the lungs. A trade name is Myleran.

Butacote – a trade name for PHENYLBUTAZONE.

Butazolidin – a trade name for PHENYLBUTAZONE.

Butazone – a trade name for PHENYLBUTAZONE.

butobarbitone – a BARBITURATE sleep-encouraging (hypnotic) drug of medium duration of action. A trade name is Soneryl.

butriptyline – a tricyclic drug used in the treatment of depression. It is taken by mouth. Possible side effects include difficulty in urination and closed-angle glaucoma. A trade name is Evadyne.

cabergoline – a dopamine agonist drug. It is used to stop unwanted milk secretion especially in infertile women. It is taken by mouth. Possible side effects include breast pain, dizziness, headache, nausea, digestive upset, palpitations and nose bleed. A trade name is Dostinex.

calcifediol – a drug similar in effect to vitamin A. A trade name is Calderol.

calcipotriol – a vitamin D analogue drug administered as an ointment for the treatment of psoriasis. Possible side effects include skin irritation and facial dermatitis. A trade name is Dovonex.

Canesten – a trade name for CLOTRIMAZOLE.

captopril – a drug used to control high blood pressure. Trade names are Acepril, Capoten, Capozide.

carbamazepine – an anticonvulsant drug. A trade name is Tegretol.

carbaryl – a drug administered in the form of a lotion or shampoo to kill head and pubic lice. A trade name is Carylderm, Clinicide.

carbenoxolone – a drug derived from liquorice root, that accelerates healing of stomach ulcers by increasing the amount of protective mucus produced by the stomach lining and by reducing the rate of acid production in the stomach. It is taken by mouth. Possible side effects include fluid retention, raised blood pressure and possibly heart failure. Trade names include Bioplex, Bioral, Pyrogastrone.

Cardura – a trade name for DOXAZOCIN.

carisoprodol – a muscle-relaxant drug. A trade name is Soprodol.

cefuroxime – a cephalosporin antibiotic drug used to treat a wide range of infections, especially of the respiratory and nervous systems. It is administered by injection. Possible side effects include digestive upsets, allergic reactions, pain at the injection site and fungal infections. A trade name is Zinacef.

centoxin – a highly purified monoclonal antibody that binds to the toxin produced by the outer cell membrane of certain bacteria (endotoxin). Endotoxin causes seriously damaging effects in the body, including toxic shock, and centoxin appears to be a major advance in the treatment of infections featuring endotoxin. It is of value only in infections with germs of the 'gram-negative' group – organisms that stain in a particular way and that are resistant to many of the commoner antibiotics.

cephalexin – a cephalosporin antibiotic drug. Trade names are Ceporex, Keflex.

cetrimide – an antiseptic drug for external use only. It is applied in the form of solutions or creams for the treatment of minor wounds, abrasions and rashes. Trade names are Cetavlex, Savlon, Vesagex.

chenodeoxycholic acid – a drug used in the treatment of cholesterol gallstones, which it gradually dissolves over a period of up to 18 months. It is taken by mouth. A common side effect is diarrhoea. Trade names are Chendol, Chenofalk, Chenocedon.

chenodiol – a drug used to dissolve gallstones. A trade name is Chenix.

chloral hydrate – a sedative and hypnotic drug used mainly for children. Trade names are Noctec, Welldorm.

chlorambucil – an anticancer drug. It is taken by mouth. Possible side effects include nausea and vomiting, loss of hair and interference with bone marrow blood cell production. A trade name is Leukeran.

chloramphenicol – an antibiotic drug, now used mainly in eye drops. Taken internally it can cause serious side effects such as optic nerve damage and a sometimes fatal interference with blood cell formation by the bone marrow (aplastic anaemia). A trade name is Chloromycetin.

chlorazepate – a benzodiazepine sedative and hypnotic. A trade name is Tranxene-SD.

chlordiazepoxide – a benzodiazepine sedative and hypnotic drug. A trade name is Librium.

chlormezanone – a benzodiazepine drug used to treat short-term anxiety states featuring severe muscle tension. It is taken by mouth. Possible side effects include nausea, dry mouth, headache, skin rashes, dizziness and jaundice. A trade name is Trancopal.

chlorothiazide – a urine-promoting (diuretic) drug used also in the treatment of high blood pressure. A trade name is Diuril.

chlorpheniramine – an antihistamine drug. Trade names are Allerchlor, Haymine, Phenetron and Piriton.

chlorpromazine – an antipsychotic and antidepressive drug. Trade names are Largactil, Ormazine, Thorazine.

chlorpropamide – an oral hypoglycaemic drug used to treat Type II diabetes. A trade name is Diabinese.

cholestyramine – a drug used to reduce high blood cholesterol. It is an anion-exchange resin that acts by binding to cholesterol in the bile to form a complex that cannot be reabsorbed and is lost in the stools. A trade name is Questran.

choline magnesium trisalicylate – an anti-inflammatory and painkilling drug used to treat rheumatoid arthritis, osteoarthritis and other joint disorders. It is taken by mouth. Possible side effects include digestive upset and allergic reactions. A trade name is Trilisate.

choline theophyllinate – a drug used in the treatment of asthma. It is similar in its action to theophylline but less irritating and can be taken by mouth.

cimetidine – a drug that blocks the action of the substance, histamine, that stimulates acid production in the stomach. It is used in cases of peptic ulcer. A trade name is Tagamet.

cinchocaine – a powerful local anaesthetic drug.

ciprofloxacin – an antibiotic drug. A trade name is Cipro.

cisplatin – an anticancer drug. Like any drug that damages cells, it has side effects. These may include nausea and vomiting, loss of hair, interference with bone marrow blood cell production and progressive kidney damage.

clavulanic acid – a drug that interferes with beta-lactamase enzymes (penicillinases) that inactivate many penicillin-type antibiotics, such as amoxycillin. Combined with the antibiotic, this drug can overcome drug resistance. Trade names of the combination: Augmentin, Timentin.

clenbuterol – a beta-adrenergic agonist drug useful in the treatment of asthma. The drug is capable of causing a considerable increase in the bulk of voluntary muscle (hypertrophy) with an increase in force and a reduction in relaxation time. It is also valuable as means of preventing the wasting (atrophy) of muscle, that has been deprived of its nerve supply, during the long period of nerve regeneration.

clindamycin – an antibiotic drug that penetrates well into bone to treat bone infection (osteomyelitis).

Clinitar – a preparation containing coal tar.

clinitest – a method of urine testing for sugar (glucose) using a tablet that is dropped into the urine in a test tube. This method gives figures for the amount of sugar present, by causing a range of colour changes from green (0.5% glucose) to orange (2% glucose). Sugar in the urine is always abnormal and usually means diabetes.

clofazimine – a drug used to treat leprosy. It is effective in controlling certain unpleasant skin reactions (erythema nodosum). A trade name is Lamprene.

clofibrate – a drug that lowers the blood cholesterol levels. A trade name is Atromid-S.

Clomid – a trade name for CLOMIPHENE.

clomiphene – a drug used to treat infertility by stimulating egg production from the ovaries (ovulation). Multiple pregnancies often result. A trade name is Clomid.

clomipramine – a tricyclic antidepressant drug that is also useful in treating illogical fears (phobias) and anxiety and obsessive states. Possible side effects include dry mouth, constipation, blurred vision and difficulty in urinating. A trade name is Anafranil.

clonazepam – a benzodiazepine drug used to control epilepsy and a form of severe facial pain (trigeminal neuralgia). A trade name is Rivotril.

clonidine – a drug that acts on arteries to lower blood pressure and control some cases of migraine and postmenopausal flushing. Stopping treatment may produce a dangerous rise in blood pressure. A trade name is Dixarit.

clorazepate – a long-acting benzodiazepine drug used to treat anxiety and depression. It is taken by mouth. Possible side effects include drowsiness, vertigo, confusion, digestive upset and skin rashes. A trade name is Tranxene.

chloroquine – one of the most important and widely-used anti-malarial drugs. Chloroquine concentrates in the red blood cells that contain malarial parasites and deprives them of nourishment. Unfortunately, many strains of malarial parasite have developed resistance to chloroquine, and other drugs must be used. Chloroquine is also useful in treating rheumatoid arthritis and lupus erythematosus, but in the doses necessary it may damage the corneas and retinas of the eyes. It is taken by mouth or injection. Possible side effects include visual loss, mental disturbances, rashes, digestive upset and bleaching of the hair. Trade names include Avloclor, Nivaquine.

clotrimazole – a drug effective against a wide range of infecting fungi including those causing thrush. It is used in the form of creams, for local application. Trade names are Canesten and Lotriderm.

clove oil – an aromatic oil distilled from the flower buds of the clove tree, used mainly by dentists as a mild antiseptic and toothache reliever. Mixed with zinc oxide, it forms a widely used temporary filling for a tooth cavity.

cloxacillin – a semisynthetic penicillin antibiotic that resists the destructive penicillinase enzymes that some germs (staphylococci) produce. The drug also resists stomach acid and so can be taken by mouth.

clozapine – a benzodiazepine antipsychotic drug used in the treatment of schizophrenia resistant to other drugs. It is taken by mouth. It is notable for the absence of tremors and repetitive movements (dyskinesias) in those taking it, but it may seriously affect white blood cell production by the bone marrow and may cause drowsiness, salivation, fatigue, dizziness, headache and urinary retention. A trade name is Clozaril.

Clozaril – a trade name for CLOZAPINE.

coal tar – a complex mixture of organic substances, especially polycyclic hydrocarbons, derived from the distillation of coal. Although the action of this mixture is not well understood, coal tar preparations are used effectively to treat various skin disorders such as eczema and psoriasis.

cobalamine – vitamin B_{12}. The specific treatment for pernicious anaemia.

Cobutolin – a trade name for SALBUTAMOL.

cocaine – the main alkaloid of the bush *Erythroxylon coca*, introduced to medicine by Sigmund Freud. Cocaine was the first effective local anaesthetic drug, but is not now widely used in medicine, having been replaced by safer drugs. It is widely used as a 'recreational' drug, producing mood elevation similar to that of AMPHETAMINE and has many undesirable and sometimes dangerous effects.

Codalgin – a trade name for a compound of CODEINE and PARACETAMOL.

Codate – a trade name for CODEINE.

codeine – an alkaloid derived from opium, used to control moderate pain, to relieve unnecessary coughing and to check diarrhoea. Codeine is not a drug of addiction and is available without prescription.

Codelix – a trade name for CODEINE.

Codesol – a trade name for PREDNISOLONE.

Codiphen – a trade name for a mixture of Aspirin and CODEINE.

Codis – a trade name for a mixture of Aspirin and CODEINE.

cod liver oil – an extract of the liver of the codfish, rich in vitamins A and D.

Cogentin – a trade name for BENZTROPINE.

colchicine – an alkaloid drug made from autumn crocus plants (*Colchicum*) and used to treat gout and to stimulate chromosome copying for genetic investigation and research.

Colifoam – a trade name for HYDROCORTISONE.

colistin – an antibiotic produced by the germ *Bacillus colistinus* and effective against *Pseudomonas aeruginosa*. It is used to sterilize the inside of the bowel and bladder and in lotions and drops for the skin and external ear.

Cologel – a trade name for METHYL CELLULOSE, used as a laxative.

Colomycin – a trade name for COLISTIN.

Combantrin – a trade name for PYRANTEL.

Comox – a trade name for CO-TRIMOXAZOLE.

Compazine – a trade name for PROCHLORPERAZINE.

Concordin – a trade name for PROTRIPTYLINE.

Conova 30 – an oral contraceptive containing ETHINYLOESTRADIOL and ethynodiol.

Contac – a trade name for a compound of ATROPINE, HYOSCINE, HYOSCYAMINE and PSEUDOEPHEDRINE used to relieve the symptoms of the common cold.

co-proxamol – an analgesic drug consisting of a combination of the drug paracetamol and the weakly narcotic drug dextro-propoxyphene. It is taken by mouth. Possible side effects include dizziness, drowsiness, nausea, vomiting and sometimes euphoria. Trade names are Distalgesic, Paxalgesic.

Corbeton – a trade name for OXPRENOLOL.

Cordarone X – a trade name for AMIODARONE.

Cordilox – a trade name for VERAPAMIL.

Corgard – a trade name for NADOLOL.

Corlan – a trade name for HYDROCORTISONE.

Coro-Nitro – a trade name for nitroglycerine (GLYCERYL TRINITRATE).

Cortaid – a trade name for HYDROCORTISONE.

Cortate – a trade name for CORTISONE.

Cortef – a trade name for HYDROCORTISONE.

Cortelan – a trade name for CORTISONE.

Cortistab – a trade name for CORTISONE.

Cosuric – a trade name for ALLOPURINOL.

Cosylan – a trade name for DEXTROMETHORPHAN.

co-trimoxazole – an effective combination of the sulphonamide drug SULPHAMETHOXAZOLE and TRIMETHOPRIM. The drug is useful in acute bronchitis, urinary infections, salmonella infections and in the treatment of typhoid carriers. Trade names are Septrin and Bactrim.

Coumadin – a trade name for WARFARIN.

cromoglycate – a drug used in allergies such as hay fever (allergic rhinitis), allergic conjunctivitis, food allergy and allergic asthma. It stabilizes the membrane of the mast cells that otherwise release histamine and other irritating substances when antibodies (IgE) and allergens (such as pollen grains) interact on their surfaces. A trade name is Opticrom.

Cuprofen – a trade name for IBUPROFEN.

curare – one of a group of resinous extracts from various South American trees *Chondodendron* and *Strychnos*. It was used as an arrow poison called 'woorara paste'. Curare acts at the junction between nerves and muscles and produces complete paralysis of all voluntary movement without having any effect on consciousness. See also CURARINE.

curarine – a poisonous alkaloid obtained from curare and used as a muscle relaxant or paralysant in general anaesthesia. It acts by competing with the nerve stimulant acetylcholine at the point at which motor nerves contact muscle fibres. The form used in anaesthesia is called tubocurarine. See also CURARE.

cyanocobalamin – vitamin B_{12}. This vitamin is necessary for the normal body usage (metabolism) of carbohydrates, fats and proteins, for blood cell formation and for nerve function. It is used in the treatment of pernicious anaemia and the intestinal malabsorption disease sprue.

Cyclidox – a trade name for DOXYCYCLINE.

Cyclimorph – a trade name for a compound of MORPHINE and CYCLIZINE.

cyclizine – an antihistamine drug used to treat nausea, vomiting and vertigo caused by disorders of the balancing mechanism in the inner ear. It is taken by mouth. Possible side effects include drowsiness, digestive upsets and allergy. A trade name is Valoid.

Cycloblastin – a trade name for CYCLOPHOSPHAMIDE.

Cyclogyl – a trade name for eye drops containing CYCLOPENTOLATE.

Cyclopane – a trade name for a compound of PAPAVERINE, ATROPINE and PARACETAMOL.

cyclopentolate – a drug used to widen (dilate) the pupils of the eyes to allow examination of the retina and other internal parts. Trade names are Mydrilate, Cyclogyl.

cyclophosphamide – an anticancer drug of the class known as alkylating agents. It acts by interfering with DNA copying. The margin between the effective dose and the dangerous dose is narrow. Side effects include loss of hair, sterility, sickness, vomiting and defective blood formation by the bone marrow. A trade name is Endoxana.

cyclopropane – a powerful, non-irritating anaesthetic gas. It has the disadvantages of being explosive and of causing heart irregularity in the presence of adrenaline.

Cyclospasmol – cyclandelate, a drug that helps to improve the blood supply to any part of the body by relaxing and widening the arteries.

cyclosporin – an important immune system suppressant drug that has greatly reduced the rate of rejection of grafted organs such as kidneys and hearts. It acts by interfering with the multiplication of the T lymphocytes that attack 'foreign' tissue. A trade name is Sandimunn.

Cyklokapron – a trade name for TRANEXAMIC ACID.

Cyprostat – a trade name for CYPROTERONE.

cyproterone – a drug that reduces the action of male sex hormones and is sometimes used to curb excessive sexuality, or sexual deviation, in men. It is also used to help in the treatment of cancer of the prostate gland. Possible side effects include depression, fatigue, breast enlargement and osteoporosis. Trade names are Androcur, Cyprostat.

Cytamen – a trade name for CYANOCOBALAMIN.

cytarabine – a drug used to treat acute leukaemia. It acts by depriving cells of substances necessary for their normal function. It causes nausea, vomiting and stomach or duodenal ulcers (local breakdown of the lining), and it interferes with the normal bone marrow blood formation.

Dactil – a trade name for PIPERIDOLATE.

Daktarin – a trade name for MICONAZOLE.

Dalacin C – a trade name for CLINDAMYCIN.

Dalmane – a trade name for FLURAZEPAM.

danazole – a synthetic progestogen drug that blocks production by the pituitary gland of the sex-gland stimulating hormone gonadotrophin. It is used to treat precocious puberty, breast enlargement in the male (gynaecomastia), excessively heavy menstrual periods (menorrhagia) and endometriosis. It is taken by mouth. Possible side effects include nausea, swelling of the feet and ankles, weight gain, oiliness of the skin and, in women, excessive growth of facial and body hair. A trade name is Danol.

Daneral-SA – a trade name for PHENIRAMINE.

Danocrine – a trade name for DANAZOLE.

Danol – a trade name for DANAZOLE.

Dantrium – a trade name for DANTROLENE.

dantrolene – a drug used to relieve muscle spasm in any spastic condition such as cerebral palsy, multiple sclerosis or spinal cord injury. It is taken by mouth or given by injection. Possible side effects include weakness, dizziness, drowsiness and vertigo. Liver damage sometimes occurs. A trade name is Dantrium.

Daonil – a trade name for GLIBENCLAMIDE.

dapsone – diaminodiphenyl sulphone. For many years this has been the standard drug to treat leprosy, but irregular use has led to the development of drug resistance. Dapsone is also used in the treatment of dermatitis herpetiformis which may be associated with coeliac disease.

Daranide – a trade name for DICHLORPHENAMIDE.

Daraprim – a trade name for PYRIMETHAMINE.

daunorubicin – an antibiotic drug that interferes with DNA synthesis and is used in the consolidation phase of the treatment of acute leukaemia. It is administered by injection. Possible side effects include loss of hair, depression of bone marrow blood cell production and heart muscle damage.

DDAVP – see desmopressin.

Deca-Durabolin – a trade name for NANDROLONE.

Decadron – a trade name for DEXAMETHASONE.

Decortisyl – a trade name for PREDNISOLONE.

Decrin – a trade name for a compound of Aspirin and CODEINE.

Deltasolone – a trade name for PREDNISOLONE.

Demerol – a trade name for PETHIDINE (meperidine).

Depo-Medrone, Depo-Medrol – trade names for METHYLPREDNISOLONE used as a long-term deposit (depot) injection.

Depo-Provera – a long-acting contraceptive, given by deposit (depot) injection, containing medroxyprogesterone.

Dequacaine – a trade name for BENZOCAINE and DEQUALINIUM in lozenge form.

Dequadin – a trade name for DEQUALINIUM in lozenge form.

dequalinium – a mild antiseptic, antibacterial and antifungal drug used locally, often in the form of lozenges. Trade names are Dequacaine, Dequadin.

Deralin – a trade name for PROPRANOLOL.

Dermacort – a trade name for a HYDROCORTISONE skin preparation.

Dermazole – a trade name for ECONAZOLE.

Dermonistat – a trade name for MICONAZOLE.

Dermovate – a trade name for clobetasol, a powerful STEROID used by local application.

DES – see DIETHYLSTILBOESTROL.

Deseril – a trade name for METHYSERGIDE.

desferrioxamine – an iron-removing agent used in iron overload conditions or iron poisoning. A trade name is Desferal.

desipramine – a tricyclic antidepressant drug. Possible side effects include dry mouth, constipation, blurred vision and difficulty in urinating. Trade names are Norpramin, Pertofran.

desmopressin – a drug used in the treatment of the disease diabetes insipidus. This is quite different from the usual kind of diabetes and is due to a shortage of a body substance (hormone) that controls urine production. Desmopressin, or DDAVP, is a long-acting substance similar to the natural pituitary hormone vasopressin. The drug is given in a nasal spray or in the form of nose drops.

desogestrel – a progestogen drug used in various oral contraceptives, often in combination with an oestrogen drug. It is taken by mouth. Possible side effects include breast enlargement, a sense of bloating, leg cramps, reduction of sexual drive and depression. Trade names are Marvelon, Mercilon.

dexamethasone – a synthetic STEROID drug used for its anti-inflammatory action and for its value in reducing waterlogging (oedema) of the brain. A trade name is Decadron.

dexamphetamine – one form of AMPHETAMINE sulphate, a drug sometimes used to treat undue sleepiness (narcolepsy), hyperactivity in children and as a waking-up drug in sleep-encouraging (hypnotic) poisoning. It is widely abused. A trade name is Dexedrine.

Dexedrine – a trade name for DEXAMPHETAMINE.

Dexmethazone – a trade name for DEXAMETHASONE.

dextromethorphan – an opium-like drug, with little useful painkilling action, used to control persistent and unproductive cough.

dextromoramide – a MORPHINE-like narcotic painkilling drug used to control severe pain. A trade name is Palfium.

dextropropoxyphene – a painkilling drug similar to methadone. The trade name is Doloxene and it is also dispensed in combination with paracetamol, as Distalgesic. Overdosage is one of the commonest causes of death by poisoning, as absorption is rapid and breathing is quickly paralysed. It is not much more effective than CODEINE and some poisoning experts think it should be withdrawn.

DF118 – dihydrocodeine tartrate, a strong painkilling drug.

Diabex – a trade name for METFORMIN.

Diabinese – a trade name for CHLORPROPAMIDE.

diacetylmorphine – HEROIN.

Diaformin – a trade name for METFORMIN.

Diamicron – a trade name for GLICLAZIDE.

diamorphine – HEROIN.

Diamox – a trade name for ACETAZOLAMIDE.

Diarrest – a combination of dicyclomine, an anti-spasm drug that relieves painful bowel cramps, and codeine phosphate.

Diatensec – a trade name for SPIRONALACTONE.

diazepam – a long-acting BENZODIAZEPINE drug used to treat severe acute anxiety, delirium tremens, epilepsy and muscle spasms. It is also used as a pre-operative medication (pre-medication). It is taken by mouth. Possible side effects include drowsiness, vertigo, low blood pressure, skin rashes, urinary retention and visual disturbances. Trade names are Valium, Diazemuls.

Dibenyline – a trade name for PHENOXYBENZAMINE.

dibromomanitol – a drug used in the treatment of chronic leukaemia.

dibromopropamidine – an antibacterial and antifungal agent for external use.

dichloralphenazone – a sleep-encouraging (hypnotic) drug used for short periods for the management of insomnia and sometimes to control delirium. It is similar to CHLORAL HYDRATE (Welldorm).

dichlorophen – a deworming drug used to remove tapeworms. A trade name is Antiphen.

dichlorphenamide – a urine-promoting (diuretic) drug with a short duration of action. It is also used in the treatment of glaucoma. A trade name is Daranide.

diclofenac – a non-steroidal anti-inflammatory drug (NSAID) used in the treatment of rheumatoid arthritis and other painful conditions. Trade names are Voltarol, Voltaren.

Diconal – a trade name for DIPIPANONE.

dicoumarol – an anticlotting (anticoagulant) drug now mainly used as a rat poison. Other more readily controllable coumarins, such as WARFARIN, are now used to control blood clotting.

Dicynene – a trade name for ETHAMSYLATE.

didanosine – a drug that interferes with the action of the enzyme reverse transcriptase by means of which the human immunodeficiency virus (HIV), the cause of AIDS, is able to convert its RNA into DNA that can incorporate itself into the human DNA and replicate in the host cell. The drug is used in the attempt to prolong the lives of sufferers from AIDS. There is no evidence that the drug can cure AIDS. It is taken by mouth. Possible side effects include damage to nerves, severe pancreatitis, nausea vomiting and headache.

didronel – a drug used to improve mineralization of bone in women suffering from osteoporosis after the menopause, especially those who have already suffered fractures. It is taken by mouth. Possible side effects include nausea, diarrhoea and a metallic taste in the mouth. A trade name is Didronel PMO (postmenopausal osteoporosis).

dienoestrol – a synthetic female sex hormone (oestrogen) drug. A trade name is Hormofemin.

diethylcarbamazine – a drug used to treat the parasitic worm diseases filariasis and onchocerciasis. The drug kills both the tiny juvenile microfilaria and the adult worms but may provoke severe reactions when the worms die. A trade name is Banocide.

diethylpropion – an AMPHETAMINE-like drug used to reduce appetite to try to help in the management of obesity. Trade names are Apisate and Tenuate Dospan.

diethylstilboestrol – DES. A synthetic female sex hormone. This is now restricted in use to the treatment of certain cancers of the prostate and the breast. If given to pregnant women it can cause cancer in the female offspring.

diflunisal – a non-steroidal anti-inflammatory drug (NSAID). It is a derivative of salicylic acid and is used to control symptoms in osteoarthritis and other painful conditions. It is taken by mouth. Possible side effects include indigestion (dyspepsia), diarrhoea, headache, dizziness, ringing in the ears (tinnitus) and skin rashes. A trade name is Dolobid.

digitalis – a drug used in the treatment of heart failure. It increases the force of contraction and produces a slower, more regular pulse. The drug is derived from the purple foxglove *Digitalis purpurea* and is usually given in the form of DIGOXIN.

digoxin – a valuable heart drug derived from the foxglove. It is the most widely used of the DIGITALIS heart drugs and is a member of the group of cardiac glycosides.

Dilantin – a trade name for PHENYTOIN.

diltiazem – a calcium channel blocker drug used to treat angina pectoris. It is taken by mouth. Possible side effects include nausea, headache, swollen ankles and a slowed heart rate. Trade names are Adizem, Britiazim, Tildiem.

Dimatab – a trade name for a compound of PARACETAMOL and PSEUDOEPHEDRINE.

Dimelor – a trade name for ACETOHEXAMIDE.

dimenhydrinate – an ANTIHISTAMINE drug used mainly to control motion sickness. The trade name is Dramamine.

dimercaprol – British Anti-Lewisite (BAL). A drug that takes up poisonous metal from the body and can be life-saving in cases of poisoning with lead, arsenic, gold, mercury, antimony, bismuth and thallium. It was developed during World War I in the course of a search for antidotes to poison war gases, particularly the arsenical Lewisite.

dimethicone – a silicone preparation used externally to retain skin moisture in cases of undue drying and to protect the skin against irritating external agencies. It is commonly used to prevent nappy rash in babies. Trade names are Siopel, Conotrane.

dimethindine maleate – an antihistamine drug used to treat hay fever, urticaria and other allergic conditions. It is taken by mouth. Possible side effects include drowsiness and slowed reactions. A trade name is Vibrocil.

Dimotane – a trade name for BROMPHENIRAMINE.

Dindevan – a trade name for PHENINDIONE.

dinoprost – a prostaglandin drug used to terminate pregnancy or to expel a fetus that has died. It is also used to treat the congenital heart disorder, persistent ductus arteriosus, in the newborn and to relieve peptic ulcer. It is taken by mouth or as a vaginal tablet or gel. A trade name is Prostin F2 alpha. Dinoprostone (trade names Prepidil, Prostin E2) is a similar drug.

Dioctyl – a trade name for DOCUSATE.

dipanone – an analgesic drug used to control moderate to severe pain. Possible side effects include drowsiness, blurred vision and a dry mouth. A trade name is Diconal.

diphenhydramine – an antihistamine drug now used mainly for its sedative properties in children and for travel sickness. A trade name is Benadryl.

diphenoxylate – a drug related to PETHIDINE and with a calming codeine-like action on the bowel. It is used to treat diarrhoea. It is sold, mixed with a little ATROPINE, under the trade name of Lomotil.

diphosphonates – a group of drugs that interfere with crystal formation and are used to relieve the symptoms of Paget's disease of bone.

diprophylline – a drug similar to AMINOPHYLLINE used to relax bronchial muscle spasm in asthma and to improve the action of the heart. A trade name is Noradran.

Diprosone – a trade name for the steroid drug BETAMETHASONE in a preparation for external use.

dipyridamole – a drug used to reduce stickiness of blood platelets and thus the risk of clot formation and stroke in people having 'mini-strokes' (transient ischaemic attacks). Aspirin is more effective, but sometimes cannot be safely taken. A trade name is Persantin.

Disalcid – salsalate, a drug of similar composition and properties to Aspirin (see ACETYLSALICYLIC ACID).

Disipal – a trade name for ORPHENADRINE.

disodium cromoglycate – see CROMOGLYCATE.

disopyramide – a drug used to prevent or control disturbances of heart rhythm. A trade name is Dirythmin.

Disprin – a trade name for Aspirin (see ACETYLSALICYLIC ACID).

Distaclor – cephaclor, one of the cephalosporin group of antibiotics.

Distalgesic – a trade name for a compound of PARACETAMOL and DEXTROPROPOXYPHENE.

Distamine – a trade name for PENICILLAMINE.

distigmine – an anticholinesterase drug used to treat myasthenia gravis. It is taken by mouth. Possible side effects include nausea, vomiting, diarrhoea and excessive salivation. A trade name is Ubretid.

disulfiram – a drug that interferes with the normal metabolism of alcohol so that a poisonous substance, acetaldehyde, accumulates. This causes flushing, sweating, nausea, vomiting, faintness, headache, chest pain and sometimes convulsions and collapse. It is used to discourage drinking, but can be dangerous. The trade name is Antabuse.

dithranol – a drug used in the treatment of the skin disease psoriasis. It interferes with cell reproduction and acts to discourage overgrowth of certain skin cells. A trade name is Exolan.

Dithrolan – a trade name for a compound of DITHRANOL and SALICYLIC ACID.

ditiocarb – the sodium salt of diethyldithiocarbamate, a powerful antioxidant and metal-removing (chelating) drug that has been used to treat immune deficiency conditions, such as AIDS. It appears to be effective in reducing the incidence of opportunistic infections and cancers in HIV positive people.

Diuresal – a trade name for FRUSEMIDE.

Diurexan – a trade name for XIPAMIDE

Dixarit – a trade name for CLONIDINE.

dobutamine – a drug used to assist in the management of heart failure. It increases the force of the contraction (inotropic agent) of the muscle of the ventricles and improves the heart output. It may be given by continuous intravenous drip. A trade name is Dobutrex.

Dolmatil – A trade name for SULPIRIDE.

Doloxene – a trade name for DEXTROPROPOXYPHENE.

domperidone – a drug used to control nausea and vomiting. An antiemetic. It acts to close the muscle ring at the upper opening of the stomach (the cardia) and to relax the ring at the lower opening (the pylorus). It is taken by mouth or suppository. Possible side effects include breast enlargement and milk secretion. Trade names are Evoxin, Motilium.

Donnalix – a mixture of ATROPINE, HYOSCINE and HYOSCYAMINE.

dopamine – a natural body catecholamine neurotransmitter derived from dopa that acts on receptors throughout the body, especially in the limbic system and extrapyramidal system of the brain and in the arteries and the heart. The effects vary with the concentration. It is used as a drug to improve blood flow to the kidneys and to increase the strength of contraction of the heart in heart failure, shock, severe trauma and blood poisoning (septicaemia). It is administered by injection in carefully controlled dosage. Possible side effects include unduly rapid heart beat and irregularity, nausea, vomiting, breathlessness, angina pectoris and kidney damage. See also dopamine receptor agonists, dopamine receptor antagonists.

Dopram – a trade name for DOXAPRAM.

Dormonoct – a trade name for LOPRAZOLAM.

Dostinex – a trade name for CABERGOLINE.

dothiepin – a tricyclic antidepressant drug. It is taken by mouth. Possible side effects include dry mouth, blurred vision, constipation and urinary retention. A trade name is Prothiaden.

doxapram – a drug that stimulates breathing and consciousness. An analeptic drug similar in its action to NIKETHAMIDE. A trade name is Dopram.

doxazosin – a selective alpha-adrenergic blocker drug used to treat high blood pressure. It is taken by mouth. Possible side effects include faintness on standing up, weakness, dizziness and headache. A trade name is Cardura.

doxepin – a tranquillizing and antidepressant drug used to treat depression, especially if associated with anxiety and agitation. It is taken by mouth. Possible side effects include urinary retention and precipitation of acute glaucoma.

doxorubicin – an antibiotic, also known as adriamycin, that interferes with the copying of DNA and thus is useful as an anticancer agent. It has many side effects including loss of hair, sickness and vomiting, interference with blood production and heart damage.

doxycycline – a tetracycline antibiotic drug that is well absorbed when taken by mouth, even after food. A trade name is Vibramycin.

Doxylin – a trade name for DOXYCYCLINE.

Dozic – a trade name for HALOPERIDOL.

Dramamine – a trade name for DIMENHYDRINATE.

Drapolene – an antiseptic skin cream containing CETRIMIDE and BENZALKONIUM chloride.

Droleptan – a trade name for DROPERIDOL.

Dromoran – a trade name for LEVORPHANOL.

droperidol – a butyrophenone antipsychotic drug that causes emotional quietening and a state of mental detachment. It is sometimes used as a pre-medication before surgery. A trade name is Droleptan.

Dryptal – a trade name for FRUSEMIDE.

Ducene – a trade name for DIAZEPAM.

Duogastrone – a trade name for CARBENOXOLONE.

Duphalac – a trade name for LACTULOSE.

Durabolin – a trade name for NANDROLONE.

Duractin – a trade name for CIMETIDINE.

Duromine – a trade name for PHENTERMINE.

Duromorph – a trade name for MORPHINE.

Dyazide – a trade name for TRIAMTERENE.

Dymadon – a trade name for PARACETAMOL.

Dynese – a trade name for an antacid combination of ALUMINIUM HYDROXIDE and magnesium hydroxate.

Dyspamet – a trade name for CIMETIDINE.

Dytac – triamterene, a urine-promoting (diuretic) drug that does not lead to loss of potassium from the body.

Ebufac – a trade name for IBUPROFEN.

ecothiopate – a powerful nerve-stimulating drug of the organo-phosphate group, used in the form of eye drops to cause pro-longed narrowing (constriction) of the pupil. The drug is useful in the treatment of some cases of glaucoma and squint. A trade name is Phospholine iodide.

econazole – an antifungal drug used to treat ringworm and thrush (candidiasis). It is administered as a cream, lotion, spray powder or vaginal pessary. Possible side effects include local irritation and burning. Trade names are Ecostatin, Pevaryl.

Ecotrin – a trade name for Aspirin.

ecstasy – a popular name for the drug 3,4-methylenedioxymet-amphetamine (MDMA), a hallucinogenic amphetamine with effects that are a combination of those of LSD and amphetamine. This drug can precipitate a persistent mental disorder with delusions of persecution (paranoid psychosis).

Edecril, Edecrin – trade names for ETHACRYNIC ACID.

edrophonium – a drug used as a test for the muscle-weakening disease myasthenia gravis. A good response to the drug usually confirms the diagnosis.

EDTA – ethylene-diamine-tetra-acetic acid. A metal-removing (chelating) drug used to treat lead poisoning or remove excess calcium.

Efcortelan – a skin ointment containing HYDROCORTISONE.

eflornithine – difluoromethylornithine (DFMO), a drug used in the treatment of African sleeping sickness (trypanosomiasis). Eflornithine appears to be as active and possibly less toxic than other drugs such as MELARSOPROL.

Efudix – a preparation of FLUOROURACIL for external application.

Elantan – a trade name for ISOSORBIDE MONONITRATE.

Elavil – a trade name for AMITRYPTYLINE.

Elyzol – a trade name for METRONIDAZOLE.

emetine – an alkaloid derived from the natural plant drug ipecacuanha, sometimes used in the treatment of infections with the single-celled parasite *Entamoeba histolytica* (amoebiasis). It has now been largely replaced by the safer METRONIDAZOLE.

enalapril – an angiotensin converting enzyme (ACE) inhibitor drug with useful action over 24 hours, used to treat high blood pressure. Trade names are Innovace, Vasotec.

Endep – a trade name for AMITRIPTYLINE.

enflurane – a volatile drug used to induce and maintain general anaesthesia. It is administered by inhalation. Possible side effects include seizures, hepatitis and kidney damage.

enolic acids – the group of non-steroidal anti-inflammatory drugs (NSAIDs) that includes PHENYLBUTAZONE, AZAPROPAZONE and PIROXICAM.

enoxacin – a quinolone antibiotic drug. It is taken by mouth.

enoximone – a drug used in heart failure to increase the force and output of the heart (an inotropic drug). It is administered by injection. A trade name is Perfan.

Epanutin – a trade name for PHENYTOIN.

ephedrine – a drug with a similar action to ADRENALINE but with a more stimulant effect on the nervous system, causing tremor, anxiety, insomnia and undue alertness. It is used to treat allergic conditions and asthma. Ephedrine nasal drops decongest a swollen nose lining.

Epilim – a trade name for SODIUM VALPROATE.

epinephrine – an alternative name for ADRENALINE. Epinephrine is the favoured medical usage in the USA, but the term 'adrenaline' is in popular use.

epoprostenol – a powerful preventive of clumping of blood particles (platelets) and thus of blood clotting. It is used with heart-lung (cardiopulmonary bypass) machines and artificial kidneys (dialysis machines) to preserve the platelets in the blood being pumped through them. Epoprostenol also widens (dilates) arteries. Also known as prostacyclin. A trade name is Flolan.

Equagesic – a trade name for a tranquillizing and painkilling drug, a compound of MEPROBAMATE, Aspirin and ethoheptazine.

Equanil – a trade name for MEPROBAMATE.

ergocalciferol – vitamin D_2. This is produced in the body by the action of ultraviolet light on the natural provitamin (ergosterol) in the skin. Vitamin D is necessary for the normal mineralization of bone. Deficiency leads to rickets in growing children and bone softening (osteomalacia) in adults.

ergometrine – an ergot derivative drug used to cause the muscle of the womb (uterus) to tighten. This can be valuable after the baby is born to close off the site of separation of the afterbirth (placenta) and prevent severe bleeding (postpartum haemorrhage). The drug is sometimes given when delivery of the baby is almost accomplished. A trade name is Syntometrine.

ergotamine – a drug that causes widened (dilated) arteries to narrow. it is thus useful in the treatment of migraine. Overdosage is dangerous. A trade name is Lingraine.

Ergotrate – a trade name for ERGOMETRINE.

Erymax – a trade name for ERYTHROMYCIN.

erythromycin – an antibiotic drug used to treat a wide range of infections. The drug is useful in people who are allergic to penicillin. Trade names are Eramycin, Erymax, EryPed, Pediamycin.

eserine – a drug sometimes used to constrict the pupil and treat a condition of raised pressure within the eye (glaucoma).

Esidrex – a trade name for HYDROCHLOROTHIAZIDE.

Esidrex-K – a trade name for HYDROCHLOROTHIAZIDE with potassium.

ethacrynic acid – a urine-promoting (diuretic) drug. A drug that acts on the tubules in the kidneys to interfere with the re-absorption of water and thus greatly increase the output of urine. A trade name is Edecrin.

ethambutol – a drug used, ideally in combination with other drugs, in the treatment of tuberculosis. Ethambutol can cause damage to the optic nerves and if persisted with after vision is affected can cause blindness. A trade name is Myambutol.

ethamsylate – a drug that reduces bleeding from small blood vessels and is used to treat excessive menstruation (menorrhagia). A trade name is Dicynene.

ethanol – the chemical name for ethyl alcohol, the main constituent of alcoholic drinks.

ethinyloestradiol – a powerful synthetic female sex hormone (oestrogen) drug that can be taken by mouth and is widely used as an ingredient in oral contraceptives. Trade names are Anovlar, Controvlar, Gynovlar, Microgynon and Minovlar.

ethionamide – a drug used in the treatment of leprosy or in cases of tuberculosis resistant to other drugs.

ethisterone – a progesterone-like drug used to treat premenstrual tension (PMT) and menstrual disorders. As NORETHISTERONE, it is also an ingredient in oral contraceptives. A trade name is Micronor.

Ethmozine – a trade name for MORACIZINE.

ethosuximide – an antiepileptic drug used in the management of absence attacks (petit mal). It has no effect against major epilepsy and may cause nausea and drowsiness. A trade name is Zarontin.

etoposide – an anticancer drug derived from a plant poison epipodophyllotoxin. It is used chiefly in the maintenance treatment of acute leukaemia after remission has been achieved and the bone marrow has recovered.

etretinate – a retinoid drug used to treat severe cases of psoriasis and other serious skin conditions, including icthyosis. It is taken by mouth. Possible side effects include nausea, vomiting, headache, liver damage, loss of hair and mood changes. A trade name is Tigason.

Eudemine – a trade name for DIAZOXIDE.

Euglucon – a trade name for GLIBENCLAMIDE.

Eugynon – an oral contraceptive containing ETHINYLOESTRADIOL and LEVONORGESTREL.

Euhypnos – a trade name for TEMAZEPAM.

Eumovate – a trade name for CLOBETASONE.

Eurax – a trade name for CROTAMITON.

evening primrose oil – a plant-derived drug used in the treatment of allergic skin disease (atopic eczema) and claimed, without good evidence, to be effective in many other conditions.

Exolan – a trade name for DITHRANOL.

factor VIII – a protein (globulin) necessary for the proper clotting of the blood. The absence of factor VIII causes haemophilia but it can be isolated from donated blood and given to haemophiliacs to control their bleeding tendency.

famciclovir – a drug closely related to a component of DNA (nucleoside analogue) used to treat shingles (herpes zoster). It is taken by mouth. Possible side effects include nausea and headache. A trade name is Famvir.

famotidine – a drug that cuts down acid secretion by the stomach. A trade name is Pepcid.

Fansidar – a trade name for a mixture of PYRIMETHAMINE and SULFADOXINE.

Farlutal – a trade name for MEDROXYPROGESTERONE.

Fasigyn – a trade name for TINIDAZOLE.

Fedrine – a trade name for EPHEDRINE.

Fefol – a trade name for a compound of FOLIC ACID and IRON.

Feldene – a trade name for PIROXICAM.

Femodene – an oral contraceptive containing ETHINYLOESTRADIOL and GESTODENE.

Fenamine – a trade name for PHENIRAMINE.

Fenbid – a trade name for IBUPROFEN.

fenbufen – a non-steroidal anti-inflammatory drug (NSAID) used to relieve inflammation and the resulting pain and stiffness. It is taken by mouth. Possible side effects include nausea, vomiting and skin rashes. A trade name is Lederfen.

fenclofenac – a non-steroidal anti-inflammatory drug (NSAID).

fenfluramine – a drug used in the management of obesity. It is thought to work by producing a sense of having eaten enough (satiety) rather than by suppressing appetite. A trade name is Ponderax.

fenoprofen – a non-steroidal anti-inflammatory drug (NSAID). It is taken by mouth. Possible side effects include digestive upset, liver and kidney damage and damage to the blood-forming cells. Trade names are Fenopron, Progesic.

fenoterol – an ADRENALINE-like drug that is valuable in the management of asthma while having comparatively little effect on the heart. Its action is similar to that of SALBUTAMOL. A trade name is Berotec.

Fenox – a trade name for nasal drops containing PHENYLEPHRINE.

fentanyl – a powerful, short-acting narcotic painkiller (analgesic). A trade name is Sublimaze.

Fentazin – a trade name for PERPHENAZINE.

Feospan – an IRON preparation.

Fergon – an IRON preparation.

Ferritard – an IRON preparation.

Ferrocap F – a trade name for a compound of FOLIC ACID and IRON.

ferrous sulphate – a bitter, greenish crystalline compound of iron used in the treatment of iron deficiency anaemia.

ferrous gluconate – an iron compound used in the treatment of iron deficiency anaemia.

Ferrum H – an IRON preparation.

Fersamal – an IRON preparation used to treat anaemia.

fibrinase – Factor XIII, a substance (enzyme) in the blood that causes side links to form between fibrin molecules so as to create a mesh of fibrin that stabilizes the blood clot. Fibrinase is also known as the fibrin-stabilizing factor. See also FACTOR VIII.

finasteride – a drug used to reduce the size of the prostate gland so as to help men suffering urinary difficulty from enlargement of the gland. Finasteride interferes with the action of a chemical activator (enzyme) that converts the sex hormone testosterone to dihydrotestosterone. It is the latter that causes the prostate to enlarge. The drug causes a significant decrease in obstruction symptoms and an increased urinary flow. Side effects of finasteride include some reduction of sex drive and decreased volume of ejaculate.

FK506 – a drug that interferes with the action of the immune system and can be used to prevent rejection of grafted organs. FK506 has also been used to treat allergic skin conditions and psoriasis. Side effects include damage to the kidneys.

Flagyl – a trade name for METRONIDAZOLE.

flavoxate – an antispasmodic drug used to treat urinary incontinence and undue frequency of urination. It is taken by mouth. Possible side effects include headache, nausea, fatigue, dry mouth, diarrhoea and blurred vision. A trade name is Urispas.

flecainide – a drug used to control irregularity of the heartbeat. It is taken by mouth. Possible side effects include nausea, vomiting, dizziness, vertigo, jaundice, visual disturbances and nerve damage. A trade name is Tambocor.

Flopen – a trade name for FLUCLOXACILLIN.

flosequinan – a new drug that acts on the smooth muscle of arteries and veins to cause both to relax and widen. This greatly reduces the load on the heart in patients with heart failure without affecting the blood supply to the various parts of the body. Side effects include headache, dizziness and palpitations. The drug is still being evaluated.

Floxapen – a trade name for FLUCLOXACILLIN.

Fluanxol – a trade name for FLUPENTHIXOL.

fluclorolone – a powerful steroid drug used externally to treat skin conditions such as psoriasis. Possible side effects include skin thinning, broken veins and stretch marks (striae). A trade name is Topilar.

flucloxacillin – a semisynthetic penicillin antibiotic, readily absorbed when taken by mouth and effective against organisms that produce penicillin-destroying enzymes (beta-lactamases). It is taken by mouth. A possible side effect is a penicillin allergic reaction. Trade names are Floxapen, Magnapen.

fluconazole – an antimycotic drug used to treat thrush (candidiasis) in any part of the body, externally or internally. It is taken by mouth. Possible side effects include nausea and vomiting. A trade name is Diflucan.

flucytosine – a drug used to treat fungal infections within the body. It can be taken by mouth and is effective against thrush (candidiasis) and against the rare internal fungus infections cryptococcosis and chromoblastomycosis. Side effects are minor.

fludrocortisone – a STEROID drug with a minor anti-inflammatory action but with a powerful sodium-retaining effect. It is useful in the treatment of Addison's disease. A trade name is Florinef.

flumazenil – a benzodiazepine antagonist drug, used in anaesthesia to reverse the effects of benzodiazepine drugs on the nervous system. It is administered by injection. A trade name is Anexate.

flunisolide – a corticosteroid drug used to treat hay fever. It is administered by metered-dose nasal spray. Possible side effects include nasal irritation. A trade name is Syntaris.

flunitrazepam – a benzodiazepine drug used for the short-term treatment of insomnia. It is taken by mouth. A trade name is Rohypnol.

fluocinolone – a steroid anti-inflammatory drug for external use. A trade name is Synalar.

fluoride – any compound containing the element fluorine, which is necessary for the healthy growth and maintenance of teeth.

Fluorigard – a trade name for FLUORIDE.

Fluoroplex – a trade name for FLUOROURACIL.

fluorouracil – a pyrimidine anticancer drug. Possible side effects include nausea and vomiting, loss of hair and interference with bone marrow blood cell production.

fluoxetine – an antidepressant drug that acts by prolonging the action of the nerve stimulator (neurotransmitter) 5-hydroxytryptamine (5HT or serotonin). It is taken by mouth. Possible side effects include nausea, vomiting, diarrhoea, insomnia, anxiety, fever, skin rash and convulsions. A trade name is Prozac.

flupenthixol – a thioxanthene antipsychotic drug used to treat schizophrenia and other psychoses. It is taken by mouth or given by injection. Possible side effects include sedation and involuntary movements. Trade names are Depixol, Fluanxol.

fluphenazine – a phenothiazine drug used to treat psychotic conditions. It can be given by injection for long-term effect. The Trade name is Modecate.

flurazepam – a benzodiazepine sedative and hypnotic. A trade name is Dalmane.

Flurets – a trade name for a fluoride preparation.

fluticasone propionate – a steroid drug used to treat bronchial asthma. It is taken by inhaler. Possible side effects include hoarseness or thrush in the mouth or throat. A trade name is Flixotide.

fluvoxamine – an antidepressant drug that acts by prolonging the action of the nerve stimulator (neurotransmitter) 5-hydroxytryptamine (5HT).

folic acid – a vitamin of the B group originally derived from spinach leaves. It is necessary for the synthesis of DNA and red blood cells. Deficiency causes megaloblastic anaemia. Folic acid is plentiful in leafy vegetables and in liver but is also produced by bacteria in the bowel and then absorbed into the circulation. Deficiency may occur after antibiotic treatment.

Folicid, Folicin – trade names for FOLIC ACID.

Fortagesic – a trade name for a compound of PARACETAMOL and PENTAZOCINE.

Fortral – a trade name for PENTAZOCINE.

foscarnet – an antiviral drug active against herpes viruses, including cytomegaloviruses, that resist ACYCLOVIR, especially in patients with AIDS. It is administered by intravenous injection. Possible side effects include thirst and increased urine output, nausea, vomiting, fatigue, headache and kidney damage.

framycetin – an antibiotic drug used externally for skin infections or as eye or ear drops. Trade names are Sofradex and Soframycin.

Framycort – a trade name for a mixture of HYDROCORTISONE and FRAMYCETIN.

Framygen – a trade name for FRAMYCETIN.

frusemide – a drug that causes an increased output of urine (a diuretic) so as to relieve the body of unwanted retained water (oedema). Frusemide acts on the kidney tubules where it interferes with chloride and sodium reabsorption from the dilute filtered urine. This prevents reabsorption of water into the blood and the result is a large volume of dilute urine. Trade names are Lasix, Frusetic and Frusid.

Frusetic – a trade name for FRUSEMIDE.

Frusid – a trade name for FRUSEMIDE.

Fucidin – a trade name for FUSIDIC ACID.

Fulcin – a trade name for GRISEOFULVIN.

Furacin – a trade name for NITROFURAZONE.

Furadantin – a trade name for NITROFURANTOIN.

furosemide – see FRUSEMIDE.

fusidic acid – a STEROID antibiotic used in the form of sodium fusidate against the penicillin-resistant (beta-lactamase-producing) germs known as staphylococci. It has no value against the similar organisms known as streptococci and is usually given in conjunction with another antibiotic such as FLUCLOXACILLIN. It is taken by mouth. Possible side effects include nausea, vomiting and skin rashes. A trade name is Fucidin.

Fybogel – a trade name for ISPHAGULA.

gamma globulin – a protein, one of the five classes of immunoglubulins (antibodies). Gamma globulin, or immunoglobulin G (IgG), is the most plentiful and provides the body's main antibody defence against infection. For this reason it is produced commercially from human plasma and used for passive protection against many infections, especially hepatitis, measles and poliomyelitis.

ganciclovir – an antiviral drug similar in composition to the DNA base guanine. It is used to treat certain severe virus infections (cytomegalovirus infections), mainly in patients with AIDS. It is administered by injection. Possible side effects include nausea, vomiting, diarrhoea, infertility, confusion, seizures and disturbance of bone marrow blood cell production. A trade name is Cymevene.

Garamycin – a trade name for GENTAMICIN.

Gastreze – a mixture of the antacids ALUMINIUM HYDROXIDE and magnesium trisilicate and the foam-dispersing agent simethicone. Used to treat indigestion and peptic ulcers.

Gastrobrom – a mixture of the antacids magnesium trisilicate, magnesium hydroxide, magnesium carbonate and chalk (calcium carbonate), used to treat indigestion and peptic ulcers.

Gastromax – a trade name for METOCLOPRAMIDE.

Gelusil – a mixture of ALUMINIUM HYDROXIDE, magnesium hydroxide and the foam-dispersing agent simethicone, used to treat indigestion and peptic ulcers.

gemeprost – a prostaglandin drug, administered as a vaginal pessary to terminate pregnancy. It causes powerful contractions of the womb at any stage of pregnancy. A trade name is Cervagem.

Genisol – a shampoo containing COAL TAR.

gentamicin – an aminoglycoside antibiotic used internally mainly for the treatment of serious infections. Otherwise, Gentamicin is used for external infections, such as those of the eye or ear. In large dosage it can cause tinnitus, deafness and kidney damage.

   – a trade name for GENTAMICIN.

Geriplex – a multivitamin preparation.

gesodene – an oestrogen/progestogen oral contraceptive. It is taken by mouth. Trade name are Femodene, Minulet.

ginseng – the root of two perennial Chinese and Korean herbs of the genus *Panax* – *P. quinquefolium* or *P. schinseng*. Ginseng is credited with the power to cure many diseases including cancer, rheumatism and diabetes, and to have powerful aphrodisiac properties. There is no evidence that the herb has any medical or other value.

glibenclamide – a sulphonylurea drug, similar in action and effect to CHLORPROPAMIDE, and used in the treatment of maturity-onset (Type II) diabetes.

gliclazide – a sulphonylurea oral hypoglycaemic drug used in the treatment of Type II diabetes. It is taken by mouth. A trade name is Diamicron.

Glimel – a trade name for GLIBENCLAMIDE.

glipizide – a sulphonylurea oral antidiabetic drug used in maturity-onset (Type II) diabetes. It operates by stimulating secretion of insulin by the pancreas and is taken by mouth. Trade names are Glibenese, Minodiab.

Glucophage – a trade name for METFORMIN.

Glucotard – a trade name for GUAR GUM.

glutaraldehyde – a substance used in solution to treat warts on the sole of the foot (plantar warts).

Glutarol – a trade name for GLUTARALDEHYDE.

glutethimide – a sedative and hypnotic drug. A trade name is Doriden.

glyceryl trinitrate – a drug highly effective in controlling the pain of angina pectoris. It is best taken in a tablet that is allowed to dissolve under the tongue and the pain is usually relieved in 2-3 minutes. Nitrates have a powerful action in widening (dilating) arteries, including the coronary arteries, thus improving the blood supply to the heart muscle.

Glyconon – a trade name for TOLBUTAMIDE.

Glymese – a trade name for CHLORPROPAMIDE.

glymidine – a sulphonylurea drug used in the treatment of non-insulin dependent diabetes. Like the other sulphonylureas, such as TOLBUTAMIDE and CHLORPROPAMIDE it is taken by mouth and reduces the blood sugar (oral hypoglycaemic drug).

gold – the precious metal, salts of which, such as sodium aurothiomalate, are used to treat rheumatoid arthritis. These are effective in slowing progress of the disease, especially in early cases, but side effects, such as mouth and tongue inflammation, itching, liver and kidney damage and blood disorders, are common.

gonadorelin – the gonadotrophin releasing hormone that prompts the production of the hormone that causes the sex glands to secrete their hormones.

gramicidin – an antibiotic used externally in ointments and creams, often in conjunction with NEOMYCIN and FRAMYCETIN. It is too poisonous for internal use.

Graneodin – an ointment containing GRAMICIDIN and NEOMYCIN.

griseofulvin – an antifungal drug derived from a *Penicillium* mould that concentrates in the outer layers of the skin and in the nails and thus is useful in the treatment of 'ringworm' (tinea) infections. Skin infections settle quickly, but tinea of the nails requires treatment for months. A trade name is Fulvicin.

Griseostatin – a trade name for GRISEOFULVIN.

Grisovin – a trade name for GRISEOFULVIN.

guanethidine sulphate – a drug used in the treatment of high blood pressure (hypertension). Trade names are Ismelin and Ganda.

guar gum – an edible natural material with the property of binding carbohydrates in the intestine and reducing the rate of absorption so as to prevent a sudden increase in blood sugar. This is helpful in diabetes.

Guarem – a trade name for GUAR GUM.

Guarine – a trade name for GUAR GUM.

Gyne-Lotremin – a vaginal preparation containing CLOTRIMAZOLE.

Gyno-Daktarin – a trade name for MICONAZOLE.

Gyno-Pevaryl – a trade name for ECONAZOLE.

Gynovlar 21 – an oral contraceptive containing ETHINYLOESTRADIOL and NORETHISTERONE.

Halcion – a trade name for TRIAZOLAM.

Haldol – a trade name for HALOPERIDOL.

Haliborange – a trade name for a preparation containing vitamins A, D and C.

haloperidol – a butyrophenone drug used in the treatment of psychiatric disorders. A trade name is Serenace.

halothane – a pungent, volatile, non-inflammable liquid anaesthetic agent. Halothane is a powerful drug that induces anaesthesia in a concentration of less than 1%. Severe liver damage occurs very occasionally, usually after a second exposure to the drug in a person who has developed an allergy to it. A trade name is Fluothane.

Hamarin – a trade name for ALLOPURINOL.

Harmogen – a trade name for PIPERAZINE.

Headclear – a trade name for a compound of PARACETAMOL, PSEUDOEPHEDRINE and CHLORPHENYRAMINE.

heparin – a complex polysaccharide organic acid found mainly in lung and liver tissue. Heparin interferes with the cascade of reactions that end in blood clotting (coagulation), and is widely used as an anticoagulant.

heroin – diamorphine. A semisynthetic drug made from MORPHINE. Its effects are the same as those of morphine, to which it is converted in the body, but it is much more soluble and is rapidly absorbed when taken by mouth. This is helpful when it is used in the control of severe terminal pain. The manufacture of diamorphine, even for medical use, is illegal in almost all countries. It is still used medically in Britain.

Herpid – a trade name for IDOXURIDINE.

hexachlorophane – a bactericidal agent used in soaps and for skin cleansing. A chlorinated phenol. A trade name is Phisohex.

Hexopal – a trade name for NICOTINIC ACID.

Hibitane – a trade name for CHLORHEXIDINE.

Histryl – a trade name for DIPHENYLPYRALINE.

Hormonin – a trade name for OESTRADIOL.

Humulin – a trade name for human INSULIN.

Hydopa – a trade name for METHYLDOPA.

hydralazine – a drug that causes arteries to widen (vasodilatation) and can be used as an adjunct to the treatment of high blood pressure (hypertension) by more conventional means. It is seldom used alone. A trade name is Apresoline.

hydrochlorothiazide – a drug used to increase the output of urine so as to relieve the body of surplus water. A thiazide urine-promoting (diuretic) drug. Trade names are Esidrex, Hydromal, Hydrosaluric, Oretic.

hydrocortisone – a natural STEROID hormone derived from the outer layer (cortex) of the adrenal gland. The drug CORTISONE is converted into hydrocortisone in the liver. Hydrocortisone has anti-inflammatory and sodium-retaining properties. A trade name is Hydrocortone.

Hydrocortisyl – a trade name for HYDROCORTISONE.

Hydromet – a trade name for a mixture of HYDROCHLOROTHIAZIDE and METHYLDOPA.

Hydrosaluric – a trade name for HYDROCHLOROTHIAZIDE.

hydroxocobalamin – vitamin B_{12}. This is the specific treatment for pernicious anaemia and is highly effective unless neurological damage has already occurred. A trade name is Cobalin-H.

hydroxyzine – an antihistamine drug used as a sedative and to control vomiting. A trade name is Atarax.

Hygroton – a trade name for CHLORTHALIDONE.

hyoscine – a drug structurally related to ATROPINE and having similar properties. Also known as Scopolamine. Trade names are Buscopan, Scopoderm.

hyoscyamine – an ATROPINE-like drug used to relax smooth muscle spasm, as in colic, and for its sedative effect.

Hypovase – a trade name for PRAZOSIN.

hypromellose – a preparation of METHYL CELLULOSE used in eye drops.

Hypurin – a trade name for a preparation of INSULIN.

ibuprofen – a painkilling (analgesic) drug with anti-inflammatory properties, useful in mild rheumatic and muscular disorders and in the relief of menstrual pain. A trade name is Brufen.

idoxuridine – a drug effective against *Herpes simplex* viruses. Idoxuridine is chemically very similar to thymidine, a substance used nutritionally by the virus, which it replaces.

ifosfamide – an alkylating agent used as an anticancer drug. It is administered by injection. Possible side effects include nausea and vomiting, loss of hair and interference with bone marrow blood cell production. A trade name is Mitoxana.

Ilotycin – a trade name for ERYTHROMYCIN.

Imferon – an IRON preparation.

imipramine – a widely used tricyclic antidepressant drug. It is taken by mouth. Possible side effects include dry mouth, constipation, blurred vision and difficulty in urinating. A trade name is Tofranil.

Imodium – a trade name for LOPERAMIDE.

Imunovir – a trade name for INOSINE PRANOBEX.

Imuran – a trade name for AZOTHIAPRINE.

Inderal – a trade name for PROPRANOLOL.

Indocid – a trade name for INDOMETHACIN.

Indolar – a trade name for INDOMETHACIN.

indomethacin – a non-steroidal anti-inflammatory drug (NSAID). Trade names are Indocid, Artracin and Indolar.

indoramin – an alpha-adrenergic blocker drug used to treat high blood pressure. It is taken by mouth. Possible side effects include drowsiness, nasal congestion, dryness of the mouth and failure of ejaculation. Trade names are Baratol, Doralese.

Indur – a trade name for ISOSORBIDE MONONITRATE.

Infacol – a trade name for DIMETHICONE.

Inflam – a trade name for IBUPROFEN.

Initard – a trade name for a slow-acting INSULIN.

inosine pranobex – a drug that enhances the efficiency of the immune system by increasing the number and activity of some of the cells responsible for attacking invading germs and cancers. Early trials in HIV-positive people suggest that the drug could delay progression to AIDS. A trade name is Imunovir.

Insulatard – a trade name for a slow-acting INSULIN.

insulin – a hormone produced by cells of the islets of Langerhans in the pancreas. Insulin eases the movement of glucose and amino acids across cell membranes into cells. It also controls the activity of certain enzymes within the cells concerned with carbohydrate, fat and protein usage. Deficiency of insulin causes diabetes. Insulin preparations may be in the 'soluble' form for immediate action or in a 'retard' form for prolonged action. Trade names are Humulin, Human monotard, Mixtard, Semitard MC.

Intal – a trade name for CROMOGLYCATE.

Intraval – a trade name for SODIUM THIOPENTONE.

Intron A – a trade name for INTERFERON.

Intropin – a trade name for DOPAMINE.

iodine – a chemical element which, in small quantities, is essential in the diet. Iodine is poisonous in excess and is sometimes used dissolved in alcoholic or a potassium iodide solution as an antiseptic. The radioactive isotope, iodine 131, is extensively used for thyroid imaging and thyroid function tests.

iodoform – a yellowish iodine compound, containing about 96% iodine, used as an antiseptic.

ipecac – a drug that promotes vomiting (an emetic) and that can be given by mouth or injection.

Ipral – a trade name for TRIMETHOPRIM.

iprindol – a tricyclic antidepressant drug. It is taken by mouth. Possible side effects include dry mouth, constipation, urinary retention, blurred vision, drowsiness and tremor. A trade name is Prondol.

iproniazid – an antidepressant drug. A trade name is Marsilid.

iron – an element essential for the formation of the vital haemoglobin of the blood. Lack of iron, or excessive loss leads to iron-deficiency anaemia. Iron, in the form of soluble salts, is provided in a variety of chemical forms for the treatment of anaemia and is usually taken by mouth. In urgent cases, or if oral therapy fails, iron salts can be given by injection.

Isogel – a trade name for ISPHAGULA.

isometheptene – a sympathomimetic drug used in the treatment of migraine. It is taken by mouth. Possible side effects include dizziness. A trade name is Midrid.

isoniazid – a drug used in the treatment of tuberculosis. The drug occasionally produces side effects such as skin rash and fever, and, rarely, nerve involvement. A trade name is Rifater.

isophane insulin – a form of INSULIN modified by adsorption on to a protein molecule protamine so as to act for up to about 12 hours with delayed onset of action. Trade names are Neuphane, Insulatard and Humulin I.

isoprenaline – an air-tube widening (bronchodilator) and heart-stimulating drug used in the treatment of asthma and heart block. It is commonly taken by inhalation from an inhaler. Trade names are Aleudrin and Medihaler-iso.

Isoptin – a trade name for VERAPAMIL.

Isopto Carpine – a trade name for PILOCARPINE eye drops in HYPROMELLOSE.

Isopto Tears – artificial tears containing HYPROMELLOSE.

isosorbide mono-, di- and trinitrate – drugs used to prevent angina pectoris and in the treatment of heart failure. They are taken by mouth. Possible side effects include headache, flushing and dizziness. Trade names are Elantan and Cedocard.

Isotard – a trade name for a preparation of INSULIN.

isotretinoin – a drug related to vitamin A and used in the treatment of severe acne that has failed to respond to other measures. It is taken by mouth. Possible side effects include dry skin, nose bleeds, eyelid and lip inflammation, pains in the muscles and joints, abdominal pain, diarrhoea and disturbances of vision. A trade name is Roaccutane.

isphagula husk – a bulking agent used to treat constipation, diverticulitis and irritable bowel syndrome. It is taken by mouth. A trade name is Fybogel.

ivermectin – a drug used to kill the tiny worms known as microfilaria in the treatment of the worm parasitic disease onchocerciasis.

Jectofer – an iron preparation given by intramuscular injection for the treatment of anaemia.

Kabikinase – a trade name for STREPTOKINASE.

kanamycin – a broad-spectrum aminoglycoside antibiotic derived from a soil fungus (actinomycete). Kanamycin is now largely replaced by GENTAMICIN. The aminoglycosides can cause deafness, tinnitus and kidney damage.

kaolin – a fine clay powder used, as a suspension in liquid, in the treatment of diarrhoea and sometimes, as a thick paste poultice, to apply local heat. The word is derived from the name of the Chinese province where it was first obtained.

Kaopectate – a trade name for KAOLIN.

Keflex – a trade name for CEPHALEXIN.

Kemadrin – a trade name for PROCYCLIDINE.

Kemicetine – a trade name for CHLOROMYCETIN.

Kenalog – a trade name for TRIAMCINOLONE.

Kest – a trade name for MAGNESIUM SULPHATE.

ketamine – a drug used to produce insensitivity to pain, and mental and emotional unconcern so that operations can be performed on conscious patients. The drug is related to PHENCYCLIDINE.

ketoconazole – an imidazole antifungal drug. Ketoconazole is absorbed into the blood from the intestine and can be used to treat internal (systemic) fungal infections as well as skin fungal infections. It can, however, damage the liver. A trade name is Nizoral.

ketoprofen – a drug in the non-steroidal anti-inflammatory (NSAID) and painkilling (analgesic) group. A trade name is Orudis.

ketotifen – a drug that prevents the release of histamine and other irritating substances from mast cells in allergic conditions. Its action is similar to that of CROMOGLYCATE but has the disadvantage of causing drowsiness. A trade name is Zaditen.

Konakion – vitamin K (phytomenadione).

labetalol – a combined alpha- and beta-blocking drug, sometimes found to be more effective in the treatment of high blood pressure (hypertension) than beta-blockers. It is taken by mouth or by intravenous infusion. Possible side effects include faintness on standing up, scalp tingling and difficulty with urination and ejaculation. Trade names are Labrocol, Trandate.

Labrocol – a trade name for LABETALOL.

lachesine – a drug sometimes used to widen (dilate) the pupils in people sensitive to ATROPINE.

lactofelicine – an antibiotic derived from the protein lactofeline in human milk. It is a single peptide and has been found to be selectively effective against various bacteria that cause diarrhoea and food poisoning, especially *Listeria* species and *Escherichia coli*.

lactulose – a disaccharide sugar that acts as a gentle but effective laxative. It is not absorbed or broken down but remains intact until it reaches the colon where it is split by bacteria and helps to retain water, thereby softening the stools. Trade names are Duphalac and Lactulose.

laetrile – a substance, amygdalin, derived from the seeds of bitter almonds, apricots and other fruit, that has been claimed to be effective in treating cancer. It is said to yield a cyanide-containing compound, mandelonitrile, under the action of enzymes said to be more plentiful in cancers than in normal tissue. There is no medically acceptable evidence that laetrile has any value in the treatment of cancer.

lamotrigine – a new anti-epilepsy drug licensed for use in patients not adequately controlled by existing drugs. It is comparatively free of side effects but these include nausea, headache, dizziness, double vision and occasional skin rashes.

Lanoxin – a trade name for DIGOXIN.

Laractone – a trade name for SPIRONOLACTONE.

Laraflex – a trade name for NAPROXEN.

Largactil – a trade name for CHLORPROMAZINE.

Larodopa – a trade name for LEVODOPA.

Lasix – a trade name for FRUSEMIDE.

Lasma – a trade name for THEOPHYLLINE.

latamoxef – a CEPHALOSPORIN antibiotic active against many Gram-negative bacilli. A trade name is Moxalactam.

Latycin – a trade name for TETRACYCLINE eye ointment.

laudanum – a solution of crude opium in alcohol (tincture of opium). The alkaloids of opium are now refined and separated and prescribed as specific drugs. Laudanum was once casually recommended for a wide range of conditions.

Ledercort – a trade name for TRIAMCINOLONE.

Lederfen – a trade name for FENBUFEN.

Lentard – a trade name for a preparation of INSULIN.

Lente insulin – a trade name for a preparation of INSULIN.

lenograstim – human blood cell colony stimulating factor produced by recombinant DNA methods (genetic engineering). It is administered by injection for the treatment of certain severe forms of anaemia. A trade name is Granocyte.

Lethidrone – a trade name for NALORPHINE.

leucovorin – a drug used to counter the otherwise fatal effects of the deliberate heavy dosage of methotrexate that is sometimes used in the treatment of leukaemia and other cancers.

Leukeran – a trade name for CHLORAMBUCIL.

levallorphan – a morphine-related drug that acts as a morphine antagonist and is used to treat morphine poisoning, especially when this is causing dangerous depression of respiration. A trade name is Lorphan.

levamisole – a deworming (anthelmintic) drug used to remove roundworms. It has also been found to have an unexpected effect in stimulating the immune system by increasing the responsiveness of certain germ-attacking cells and encouraging the activity of scavenging (phagocyte) cells. It is effective in rheumatoid arthritis. The drug is taken by mouth. Possible side effects include joint pains and arthritis and these limit its use.

levodopa – a drug used to control the symptoms of Parkinsonism. Trade names are Dopar, Larodopa.

levonorgestrel – a synthetic female sex hormone similar in effect to progesterone and used mainly as an oral contraceptive. It is taken by mouth. Possible side effects include water retention with ankle swelling and weight gain, irregular vaginal bleeding, breast tenderness, nausea and headache. Trade names are Microval, Norgeston.

Levophed – a trade name for NORADRENALINE.

Libanil – a trade name for GLIBENCLAMIDE.

Librax, Libraxin – trade names for a compound of CHLORDIAZEPOXIDE and the ATROPINE-like, sympathetic nervous system blocking drug clidinium bromide.

Librium – a trade name for CHLORDIAZEPOXIDE.

Lidocaine – a trade name for LIGNOCAINE or Xylocaine.

Lidothesin – a trade name for LIGNOCAINE or Xylocaine.

lignocaine – a widely used local anaesthetic drug which is also used by intravenous injection in the treatment or prevention of acute disorders of heart rhythm such as the severe slowing of ventricular tachycardia and the deadly ventricular fibrillation – a form of cardiac arrest.

Limbritol – a trade name for a compound of AMITRIPTYLINE and CHLORDIAZEPOXIDE.

Lincocin – a trade name for LINCOMYCIN.

lincomycin – an antibiotic drug used to treat penicillin-resistant infections. A trade name is Lincocin.

lindane – an insecticide drug used externally to kill parasites such as lice and the scabies mite *Sarcoptes scabei*. It is applied externally as a lotion or cream. Possible side effects include skin irritation and rashes, but these are rare. Trade names are Quellada, Lorexane.

Lingraine – a trade name for ERGOTAMINE.

Lioresal – a trade name for BACLOFEN.

Liquifilm Tears – artificial tears containing polyvinyl alcohol.

Liskonum – a trade name for LITHIUM.

Litarex – a trade name for LITHIUM.

Lithicarb – a trade name for LITHIUM.

lithium – an element, the lightest known solid. It is used in the citrate or carbonate form for the control of manic depressive states. A trade name is Eskalith. Lithium is also used as the succinate in ointments for the treatment of certain forms of dermatitis and in shampoos for the control of dandruff. Trade names are Liskonum, Litarex, Lithicarb.

lobeline – a mixture of alkaloids with action similar to nicotine. Lobeline is derived from plants of the *Lobelia* genus and has been used as a respiratory stimulant, but is of little medical importance.

Locoid – a trade name for HYDROCORTISONE.

Loestrin – an oral contraceptive containing ETHINYLOESTRADIOL and NORETHISTERONE.

lofepramine – a drug used in the treatment of depression. It is taken by mouth or injection. Possible side effects include flushing, sweating, dryness of the mouth, blurred vision, difficulty in passing urine and drowsiness. A trade name is Gamanil.

Logynon – an oral contraceptive containing ETHINYLOESTRADIOL and LEVONORGESTREL.

Lomotil – a mixture of DIPHENOXYLATE and ATROPINE.

lomustine – an anticancer drug. It is taken by mouth. Possible side effects include nausea and vomiting, loss of hair and interference with bone marrow blood cell production. Trade names are CCNU, CeeNU.

loperamide – a synthetic narcotic-type drug used to control mild diarrhoea. A trade name is Imodium.

loprazolam – a long-acting benzodiazepine drug taken by mouth. Possible side effects include addiction and rebound insomnia. A trade name is Loprazolam.

Lopresor – a trade name for METOPROLOL.

lorazepam – a benzodiazepine tranquillizer drug similar to Valium (DIAZEPAM). A trade name is Ativan.

lorcainide – a drug used to treat irregularity of the heartbeat,

lormetazepam – a benzodiazepine drug of intermediate duration of action, used to treat insomnia. It is taken by mouth. Possible side effects include confusion, light-headedness, loss of balance and skin rashes.

Losec – a trade name for the proton pump inhibitor drug OMEPRAZOLE.

Lotremin – a trade name for CLOTRIMAZOLE.

lovastatin – an HMG-CoA reductase inhibitor cholesterol-lowering drug. A trade name is Mevacor.

Ludiomil – a trade name for MAPROTILINE.

Lugacin – a trade name for GENTAMICIN.

Madopar – a proprietary drug containing a mixture of a DOPAMINE precursor and an inhibitor of the enzyme, dopa decarboxylase, that breaks down dopamine. Madopar is used to treat the form of Parkinsonism that sometimes follows encephalitis (post-encephalitic Parkinsonism). It is taken by mouth. Possible side effects include nausea, vomiting, loss of appetite, fainting on standing up and involuntary movements.

Magnapen – a mixture of the penicillin antibiotics AMPICILLIN and FLUCLOXACILLIN.

magnesium carbonate – a mild antacid drug used to treat indigestion (dyspepsia). A trade name is Actonorm.

magnesium hydroxide – an antacid and laxative drug. A trade name is Milk of Magnesia.

magnesium sulphate – a drug used by mouth or by enema to treat constipation; by local application in a paste or poultice to draw water from wounds; and by injection to treat magnesium deficiency. Trade names are Kest, Magnoplasm.

magnesium trisilicate – a drug used as an antacid in the treatment of indigestion (dyspepsia). A trade name is Actonorm.

Magnoplasm – a trade name for MAGNESIUM SULPHATE.

Maloprim – a trade name for a compound of PYRIMETHAMINE and DAPSONE used in the treatment of malaria in the hope of eliminating the liver cycle (exoerythrocytic cycle) and thus preventing recurrences.

maprotiline – an antidepressant drug. A trade name is Ludiomil.

Marcaine – a trade name for the long-acting local anaesthetic drug BUPIVACAINE. The effect lasts for about four hours.

Marevan – a trade name for the anticoagulant drug WARFARIN.

Marplan – a trade name for the monoamine oxidase inhibitor (MAOI) antidepressant drug isocarboxazid.

Marvelon – an oral contraceptive containing ETHINYLOESTRADIOL and the progestogen drug DESOGESTREL.

Marzine – a trade name for the antihistamine and antiemetic drug CYCLIZINE.

Maxidex – a trade name for the steroid drug DEXAMETHASONE in the form of eye drops.

Maxolon – a trade name for the antiemetic and antinausea drug METOCLOPRAMIDE.

mebanazine – a monoamine oxidase inhibitor (MAOI) drug used in the treatment of severe depression.

mebendazole – an anthelmintic drug used to get rid of round-worms, hookworms, threadworms and whipworms.

mebeverine – an antispasmodic drug used to treat abdominal pain and cramps such as those occurring in the irritable bowel syndrome. It is taken by mouth. A trade name is Colofac.

mecillinam – a penicillin-type antibiotic. It is taken by mouth. Possible side effects include allergic reactions and digestive upset. A trade name is Selexidin.

meclozine – an anti-nerve-stimulating drug that has an inhibitory action on the vomiting centre of the brain and is used to prevent motion sickness. A trade name is Bonamine.

medazepam – a short-acting benzodiazepine sedative drug used as a sleep-encouraging (hypnotic). A trade name is Nobrium.

Medomet – a trade name for the antihypertensive drug METHYLDOPA.

Medrone – a trade name for the steroid drug METHYLPREDNISOLONE.

medroxyprogesterone – a progestogen drug that can be taken by mouth and is used to treat menstrual disorders and the pre-menstrual syndrome (PMS). A trade name is Provera.

mefenamic acid – a non-steroidal anti-inflammatory drug (NSAID) painkilling drug.

mefloquine – a drug used in the prevention and treatment of malaria. It is taken by mouth. A trade name is Lariam.

mefruside – a thiazide-like diuretic drug. It is taken by mouth. Possible side effects include indigestion (dyspepsia) and nausea. A trade name is Baycaron.

melarsan oxide – a preparation of arsenic used, in conjunction with other drugs that reduce its toxicity, to treat African sleeping sickness.

melarsoprol – a combination of MELARSAN OXIDE and DIMERCAPROL used to treat sleeping sickness (trypanosomiasis) by killing the *Trypanosoma gambiense*. The drug is highly effective but must be used with caution because of sometimes dangerous side effects such as severe damage to the nervous system.

Melleril – a trade name for the phenothiazine antipsychotic drug THIORIDAZINE.

melphalan – a drug used in the treatment of excess haemoglobin in the blood (polycythaemia vera), chronic leukaemia and myeloma.

meperidine – another name for PETHIDINE.

mepivacaine – a local anaesthetic drug. It is administered by injection.

Meprate – a trade name for MEPROBAMATE.

meprobamate – a sedative and tranquillizing drug. Trade names are Equanil, Meprospan, Miltown.

meptazinol – a synthetic opium-like and narcotic painkiller. A trade name is Meptid.

Meptid – a trade name for MEPTAZINOL.

mercaptopurine – a drug used in combination with others in the treatment of leukaemia and other forms of cancer.

mesterolone, mestrolone – a synthetic male sex hormone drug similar to testosterone. It is used to treat loss of sexual interest (loss of libido) and failure of full development of the secondary sexual characteristics due to sex hormone deficiency. It is taken by mouth. Possible side effects include prolonged erections (priapism), liver damage or even liver cancer. A trade name is Pro-viron.

metaraminol – a sympathomimetic alpha adrenoreceptor agonist drug used to treat severe allergic reactions (anaphylactic shock). It is administered by injection. A trade name is Aramine.

Metatone – a trade name for a mixture of vitamin B_1 (thiamine) and glycerophosphates.

metformin – a drug used in the treatment of maturity-onset diabetes (non-insulin-dependent diabetes). The drug may be dangerous to those with liver or kidney disease or a high alcohol intake. A trade name is Orabet.

methadone – a synthetic narcotic painkilling (analgesic) drug with properties similar to those of MORPHINE. It is also used as a substitute for HEROIN in attempts to manage addiction, but is widely abused. A trade name is Dolophine.

methimazole – a drug used in the treatment of overactivity of the thyroid gland. It is effective in reducing thyroid activity but may cause a dangerous loss of white blood cell production (agranulocytosis). A sore throat is a warning symptom.

Methixene – an anti-nerve-stimulating (anticholinergic) drug used to control the symptoms of Parkinson's disease. It is taken by mouth. Possible side effects include nausea, digestive upset, fatigue and weakness. A trade name is Tremonil.

Methoblastin – a trade name for METHOTREXATE.

methotrexate – a drug that interferes with cell function and with the normal operation of the immune system. It is used to treat cancer and help in the treatment of rheumatoid arthritis. It acts by interfering with the body's normal usage of FOLIC ACID.

methoxyflurane – a volatile general anaesthetic drug. It is administered by inhalation. Possible side effects include liver damage and dangerously high fever.

methyl cellulose – an inert and indigestible substance that has been used to bulk out meals in the hope of achieving weight loss. It is also used as a laxative and in artificial tears.

methylcysteine – a mucous-dissolving drug used to help to relieve the symptoms of chronic bronchitis and to reduce the production of excessively sticky mucus. It is taken by mouth. Possible side effects include digestive upset.

methyldopa – a drug used to treat high blood pressure. A trade name is Aldomet.

methylphenobarbitone – a barbiturate drug used for the long-term control of epilepsy. The drug is reduced to phenobarbitone in the body. It is taken by mouth. Possible side effects include drowsiness, dizziness, headache, confusion and sometimes, paradoxically, over-excitement. A trade name in Prominal.

methylprednisolone – a synthetic corticosteroid drug used to prevent graft rejection after organ transplantation and, often as a depot injection, to treat inflammation. Trade names are Depo-Medrone, Medrone, Solu-Medrone.

methylprogesterone – a synthetic drug similar to the female sex hormone progesterone. It is used to treat excessive menstruation, some cases of infertility, abnormal placement of womb lining (endometriosis), and some cases of breast cancer in post-menopausal women. It is taken by mouth. Possible side effects include weight gain, breast pain and milk secretion. A trade name is Provera.

methyltestosterone – a male sex hormone drug sometimes used to treat the severe itching caused by cirrhosis of the liver. A trade name is Android.

methylxanthine derivatives – drugs such as THEOPHYLLINE and AMINOPHYLLINE used in the treatment of asthma.

methysergide – an ergot derivative drug used to treat resistant cases of migraine. Its use carries some risk of interfering with the blood supply to part of the brain.

metoclopramide – an antivomiting (antiemetic) drug also useful in the control of severe heartburn (reflux oesophagitis) in hiatus hernia.

Metox – the antivomiting (antiemetic) drug METOCLOPRAMIDE.

metrifonate – an organophosphorus drug used to kill the parasitic worms in schistosomiasis, especially *Schistosoma haematobium*.

Metrogyl – a trade name for METRONIDAZOLE.

Metrolyl – a trade name for METRONIDAZOLE.

metronidazole – an antibiotic drug effective against *Trichomonas vaginalis* and *Entamoeba histolytica* as well as many other organisms. It is especially useful in the treatment of amoebic dysentery and amoebic liver abscesses as well as in anaerobic infections. A trade name is Flagyl.

Metrozine – a trade name for METRONIDAZOLE.

metyrapone – a drug that interferes with the production of the hormone aldosterone and used in the treatment of Cushing's syndrome. It is taken by mouth. Possible side effects include nausea, vomiting, low blood pressure and allergic reactions. A trade name is Metopirone.

mexiletine – an anti-arrhythmic drug used in the treatment or prevention of severe heart irregularity arising in the lower chambers (ventricles). It is taken by mouth. Possible side effects include digestive upset and low blood pressure with faintness. A trade name is Mexetil.

miconazole – an imidazole antifungal drug. It can be taken by mouth or given by intravenous injection in severe systemic fungal infections. A trade name is Monistat.

Microgynon – a low-dose oral contraceptive pill containing ETHINYLOESTRADIOL and levonorgestrel.

Micronor – a low-dose oral contraceptive pill containing NORETHISTERONE.

Microvar – a low-dose oral contraceptive containing the progestogen drug levonorgestrel.

Midamor – a trade name for AMILORIDE.

midazolam – a benzodiazepine drug used as a sedative for minor surgery, as a premedication and to induce general anaesthesia. It is administered by injection. Possible side effects include headache, dizziness, hiccup and difficulty in breathing. A trade name is Hypnovel.

mifepristone – the drug RU486, known as the 'abortion pill', that acts by blocking the action of PROGESTERONE which is essential to maintain pregnancy. A second drug, one of the prostaglandins, has to be taken within 48 hours to complete the expulsion of the fertilized egg. The method is said to be 95% effective.

Migral, Migril – trade names for a compound of the antimigraine drugs ERGOTAMINE, CAFFEINE and CYCLIZINE.

Migranol – a trade name for a compound of PARACETAMOL, ATROPINE, PAPAVERINE and nicotinic acid.

Minihep – a trade name for the anticoagulant drug HEPARIN.

Minocin – a trade name for the tetracycline antibiotic drug minocycline.

minoxidil – an artery-widening (vasodilator) drug used in the treatment of high blood pressure (hypertension). The drug has acquired a partially-justified reputation as a hair-restorer. Trade names are Regaine, Rogaine.

Mintezol – a trade name for THIABENDAZOLE.

misoprostol – a prostaglandin E_1 drug used in the prevention and treatment of peptic ulcer caused by non-steroidal anti-inflammatory drugs (NSAIDs). It is taken by mouth. Possible side effects include nausea, vomiting, diarrhoea and abdominal pain. Trade names are Cytotec, Napratec.

mithramycin – a drug that reduces bone metabolism and can be useful in the treatment of Paget's disease and excessive blood calcium (hypercalcaemia).

mitotane – a drug used to treat cancer of the adrenal glands. It is taken by mouth. Possible side effects include nausea, vomiting and skin rashes.

Mixtard – a trade name for a preparation of INSULIN with a prolonged action.

Mobilan – a trade name for INDOMETHACIN.

moclobemide – a new antidepressant drug of a class known as reversible inhibitors of monoamine oxidase type A. Existing monoamine oxidase inhibitors can cause severe reactions when cheese or other tyramine-containing foods are eaten by patients taking them. These effects are less likely with reversible inhibitors.

Modecate – a trade name for the tricyclic antipsychotic drug FLUPHENAZINE.

Moduretic – a potassium-sparing thiazide diuretic drug.

Mogadon – a trade name for NITRAZEPAM.

Monistat – a trade name for a cream containing MICONAZOLE.

Monophane – a trade name for a preparation of INSULIN.

Monotard – a trade name for a preparation of INSULIN.

moracizine – a drug used to treat life-threatening irregularity of the heartbeat (arrhythmia). It is taken by mouth. Possible side effects include nausea, dizziness, worsening of the arrhythmia and heart failure. It is used only in cases in which the risks are thought to be justified.

morphine – a powerful narcotic painkilling (analgesic) drug used to control severe pain and to relieve anxiety after severe injury. It is also an effective cough suppressant. It is administered by injection or by mouth. Possible side effects include nausea, vomiting, constipation, discouragement of breathing, coma or death from overdose and, sometimes, addiction. Trade names are Cyclimorph and Sevredol.

Motillium – the antivomiting (antiemetic) drug DOMPERIDONE.

Motrin – a trade name for IBUPROFEN.

Moxacin – a trade name for AMOXYCILLIN.

Mucomyst – a trade name for ACETYLCYSTEINE.

Myadec – a trade name for a multivitamin and mineral preparation.

Myambutol – a trade name for ETHAMBUTOL.

Mycifradin – a trade name for NEOMYCIN.

Myciguent – a trade name for an ointment containing the antibiotic NEOMYCIN.

Mycostatin – a trade name for NYSTATIN.

Mydriacyl – a trade name for eye drops containing TROPICAMIDE.

Mygdalon – a trade name for the antivomiting (antiemetic) drug METOCLOPRAMIDE.

Mylanta – a trade name for a compound of the antacid drugs ALUMINIUM HYDROXIDE and magnesium hydroxide and the antifoaming preparation SIMETHICONE.

Myleran – a trade name for BUSULPHAN.

Mynah – a trade name for the anti-tuberculosis drug ETHAMBUTOL.

Myoquine – a trade name for QUININE.

Mysoline – the anti-epilepsy (anti-convulsant) drug primidone.

Mysteclin – a mixture of the antifungal drug NYSTATIN and the antibiotic TETRACYCLINE.

nabilone – a cannabinoid drug, related to marijuana, used to control severe nausea and vomiting. It is thought to act on opiate receptors in the nervous system. It is taken by mouth. A trade name is Cesamet.

nadolol – a beta-blocker drug. It is taken by mouth. Possible side effects include sleep disturbance, tiredness, digestive upset, cold hands and feet, asthma and undue slowing of the heart. A trade name is Corgard.

naftidrofuryl – a drug that acts to relax the muscles in the walls of arteries so that the vessels widen and allow more blood to flow through to the brain, the muscles and other parts of the body. It is taken by mouth. Possible side effects include nausea and abdominal pain. A trade name is Praxilene.

Nalcrom – a trade name for CROMOGLYCATE.

nalidixic acid – a quinolone antibiotic drug used for urinary infections. It is taken by mouth. Possible side effects include nervous system upsets, skin rashes, visual disturbances and convulsions. A trade name is Negram.

nalorphine – a narcotic antagonist drug.

naloxone – a narcotic antagonist drug, chemically related to MORPHINE, and used as an antidote to narcotic poisoning. A trade name is Narcan.

naltrexone – a narcotic antagonist drug used in the maintenance treatment of heroin and other opioid-dependent patients. It is taken by mouth. A trade name is Nalorex.

nandrolone – a male sex hormone with muscle-building (anabolic) properties. The drug is sometimes used also to stimulate blood cell production in aplastic anaemia. It is administered by injection. Possible side effects include heart enlargement, oedema and virilization in women. A trade name is Deca-Durabolin.

naphazoline – an ADRENALINE-like drug that causes small blood vessels to constrict and thus reduces congestion in mucous membranes. It may be taken as a nasal spray. A trade name is Antistin Privine

Naprogesic – a trade name for NAPROXEN.

Naprosyn – a trade name for NAPROXEN.

naproxen – a non-steroidal anti-inflammatory drug (NSAID). Trade names are Naprogesic, Naprosyn.

Narcan – a trade name for NALOXONE.

Nardil – the antidepressant drug phenelzine.

Narphen – the narcotic painkilling drug phenazocine.

Natulan – the anticancer drug procarbazine.

Navidrex – a trade name for the thiazide urine-promoting (diuretic) drug cyclopenthiazide.

Nazen – a trade name for NAPROXEN.

nedocromil – an anti-inflammatory drug used to treat bronchitis, bronchial asthma, late-onset asthma and exercise-induced asthma. It is administered by metered dose aerosol inhaler. Possible side effects include nausea and brief headaches. A trade name is Tilade.

Nembudeine – a trade name for a compound of the painkillers PARACETAMOL and CODEINE and the sedative PENTOBARBITONE.

Nembutal – a trade name for PENTOBARBITONE.

Neo Cortef – a trade name for a preparation, for external use, containing the anti-inflammatory drug HYDROCORTISONE and the antibiotic NEOMYCIN.

Neo-Hycor – a trade name for eye preparations containing the anti-inflammatory drug HYDROCORTISONE and the antibiotic NEOMYCIN.

Neo-Medrol – a trade name for a skin preparation containing the steroid drug METHYLPREDNISOLONE and the antibiotic NEOMYCIN.

Neo-Mercazole – a trade name for CARBIMAZOLE.

neomycin – an aminoglycoside antibiotic drug derived from a fungal *Streptomyces fradiae*. Neomycin can be given by mouth to destroy organisms in the bowel or can be used in solution to irrigate the bladder. It is poorly absorbed into the bloodstream. It is much too poisonous to be given by injection and can have seriously damaging effects on hearing and on the kidneys. The drug is widely used as a surface application in ointments.

Neophryn – a trade name for PHENYLEPHRINE.

Neoplatin – a trade name for CISPLATIN.

neostigmine – a drug used in the treatment of the muscle-weakening disease myasthenia gravis.

Nepenthe – a trade name for MORPHINE.

Nephril – the thiazide urine-promoting (diuretic) drug polythiazide.

Netilin – a trade name for NETILMICIN.

Neuroremed – a trade name for TRYPTOPHAN.

niacin – one of the B group of vitamins. Also called nicotinic acid. Niacin is present in liver, meat, grains, beans and peas. It is a constituent of coenzymes involved in oxidation-reduction reactions. Deficiency causes pellagra. Niacin is sometimes used in the treatment of high blood cholesterol levels.

nicardipine – a calcium antagonist drug used to treat long-term stable angina pectoris. It is taken by mouth. Possible side effects include nausea, chest pain, dizziness, headache, flushing, a feeling of warmth and palpitations. A trade name is Cardene.

niclosamide – an anthelmintic drug used to remove tapeworms. It is taken by mouth. Unlike earlier treatments, it is free from side effects. A trade name is Yomesan.

Nicorette – chewing gum containing nicotine (see Chapter 5) used to assist in giving up smoking. Nicotine is also available in skin patches for transdermal administration under the trade name Nicotinell.

nicotinamide – see NIACIN.

nicotinic acid – see NIACIN.

Nidazol – a trade name for METRONIDAZOLE.

nifepidine – a drug used to control the symptoms of angina pectoris. It has a powerful effect in widening (dilating) arteries, including the coronary arteries, and this improves the blood supply to the heart muscle. The drug, however, causes flushing, headache, skin itching and dizziness. It is often used in combination with a beta-blocker. A trade name is Adalat.

nifurtimox – a drug used in the treatment of South American trypanosomiasis (Chagas' disease). The drug is effective against the causal agent *Trypanosoma cruzi* but its use is associated with side effects such as nausea, vomiting, loss of appetite, abdominal pain, muscle and joint aches, headache and vertigo.

nikethamide – a 'waking-up' (analeptic) drug used to treat light coma, drowsiness and inadequate depth of respiration. It can raise the level of consciousness in comatose patients so that they can be encouraged to cough and bring up bronchial secretions. It is taken by mouth or injection. Possible side effects include nausea, vomiting, rapid and irregular heartbeat, dizziness, restlessness, tremor and convulsions.

Nilstat – a trade name for the antifungal drug NYSTATIN.

niridazole – a drug used in the treatment of the worm parasite disease schistosomiasis. It is highly effective against the *Haematobium* variety but because of its side effects it has been largely replaced by other drugs such as PRAZIQUANTEL.

Nitradisc – a trade name for a preparation of the angina-relieving drug GLYCERYL TRINITRATE.

Nitrados – a trade name for NITRAZEPAM.

nitrazepam – a long-acting benzodiazepine sleep-encouraging (hypnotic) drug, widely used to promote sleep in insomnia. A trade name is Mogadon.

Nitro-bid – a trade name for a preparation of the angina-relieving drug GLYCERYL TRINITRATE.

Nitrocine – a trade name for GLYCERYL TRINITRATE.

nitrofurantoin – an antibacterial drug used to treat urinary infections. It is taken by mouth. Possible side effects include digestive upsets, lung disturbances with coughing of blood, peripheral nerve upsets and allergic reactions. Trade names are Furadantin, Macrobid, Macrodantin.

nitrofurazone – a drug used in the treatment of sleeping sickness (African trypanosomiasis).

nitrogen mustard – a drug used in the treatment of cancer. Nitrogen mustard reacts with tumour DNA to prevent it from replicating.

nitroglycerine – a drug widely used to relieve the symptoms of angina pectoris. It is commonly taken in a tablet allowed to dissolve under the tongue. Trade names are Nitrolingual, Nitronal.

Nitrolate – a trade name for a preparation of the angina-relieving drug GLYCERYL TRINITRATE.

Nitrolingual – a trade name for NITROGLYCRINE.

Nitronal – a trade name for NITROGLYCERINE.

nitroprusside – a drug used in the emergency treatment of high blood pressure. It is given by controlled infusion into a vein and is the most effective known means of reducing dangerously high pressure. It must, however, be used with great care and its effects closely monitored. Possible side effects include nausea, vomiting, headache, palpitations, sweating and chest pain.

Nivaquine – a trade name for CHLOROQUINE.

Nizoral – a trade name for KETOCONAZOLE.

Nobrium – a trade name for MEDAZEPAM.

Nolvadex – a trade name for TAMOXIFEN.

norethandrolone – a synthetic anabolic steroid similar in chemical structure to TESTOSTERONE.

norethisterone – a progestogen drug commonly used alone, or in combination with an oestrogen, as an oral contraceptive. A trade name is Gynovlar.

Norflex – a trade name for ORPHENADRINE.

Norgesic – a trade name for ORPHENADRINE.

Normison – a trade name for TEMAZEPAM.

Nortap – a trade name for NORTRIPTYLINE.

nortriptyline – a tricyclic antidepressant drug. It is taken by mouth. Possible side effects include constipation, blurred vision, dryness of the mouth and difficulty in urinating. A trade name is Aventyl.

Norval – a trade name for the antidepressant drug myaserin.

novobiocin – an antibiotic drug formerly of importance in the treatment of infections with bacteria resistant to other antibiotics but now largely replaced by beta-lactamase resistant penicillins.

Novocain – a trade name for the local anaesthetic drug PROCAINE.

Nozinan – a trade name for the antipsychotic drug methotrimeprazine.

Nubain – a trade name for the narcotic painkilling drug nalbuphine.

Nuelin – a trade name for THEOPHYLLINE.

Nulacin – a trade name for a mixture of calcium carbonate and MAGNESIUM TRISILICATE. An antacid preparation.

Nupercaine – a trade name for the local anaesthetic drug CINCHOCAINE.

Nurophen – a trade name for IBUPROFEN.

Nyspes – a trade name for NYSTATIN.

Nystan – a trade name for NYSTATIN.

nystatin – a drug used in the treatment of fungus infections, such as thrush. Nystatin is used for external infections only as it is not absorbed when given by mouth and is too poisonous to be given by injection. Trade names are Mycostatin, Nyspes, Nystan.

Ocusert – a device inserted behind the lower eyelid that releases PILOCARPINE into the tear film for the treatment of glaucoma.

ofloxacin – a quinolone antibiotic drug used to treat urinary tract and sexually-acquired infections It is taken by mouth or given by injection. Possible side effects include nausea, vomiting, skin rashes, nervous system disturbances and convulsions. A trade name is Tarivid.

olsalazine – an Aspirin-like drug (salicylate) used to treat mild ulcerative colitis. It is taken by mouth. Possible side effects include nausea, vomiting, headache, joint pain and skin rashes. A trade name is Dipentum.

omeprazole – the first of a new class of proton pump inhibitor drugs used to control the production of stomach acid and treat stomach and duodenal ulcers (cratering of the lining) and especially the serious ulcerating condition, the Zollinger-Ellison syndrome. Omeprazole can be effective in cases that have failed to respond to histamine receptor blocker drugs such as RANITIDINE. The drug is long-acting and need only be taken once a day. Trade names are Losec, Prilosec.

Omnopon-scopolomine – a trade name for a compound of HYOSCINE and PAPAVERETUM.

ondansetron – a drug used for the control of severe nausea and vomiting. Ondansetron works by opposing the action of the nerve activator (neurotransmitter) serotonin. It is mainly used to relieve the effects of some anticancer drugs and to prevent postoperative vomiting.

Opilon – a trade name for THYMOXAMINE.

Opticrom – a trade name for CROMOGLYCATE.

Orabet – a trade name for the antidiabetic drug METFORMIN.

Oradexon – a trade name for DEXAMETHASONE.

Orap – the antipsychotic and movement disorder drug PIMOZIDE.

Orbenin – a trade name for CLOXACILLIN.

oroxine – the thyroid hormone THYROXINE.

orphenadrine – a drug used to relieve muscle spasm, especially in Parkinson's disease. A trade name is Disipal.

Orudis – a trade name for KETOPROFEN.

Otrivine – a trade name for the decongestant drug XYLOMETAZOLINE.

oxamniquine – a drug used in the treatment of the parasitic worm disease schistosomiasis.

oxantel – a drug used in the treatment of *Trichuris* worm infections.

oxatomide – an antihistamine drug used to treat hay fever. It is taken by mouth. Possible side effects include drowsiness and slowed reactions. A trade name is Tinset.

oxazepam – a benzodiazepine tranquillizing drug. A trade name is Serenid.

oxprenolol – a beta-blocker drug used to treat angina pectoris, high blood pressure (hypertension) and disorders of heart rhythm. Possible side effects include sleep disturbance, tiredness, digestive upset, cold hands and feet, asthma and undue slowing of the heart. A trade name is Trasicor.

oxymetazoline – a sympathomimetic drug used to treat nasal congestion. It is administered as a nasal spray. Possible side effects include irritation of the nose, headache, fast pulse and insomnia. A trade name is Afrazine.

oxymetholone – an anabolic steroid drug with similar actions to TESTOSTERONE. A trade name is Anadrol-50.

Oxymycin – a trade name for OXYTETRACYCLINE.

oxyphenbutazone – a non-steroidal anti-inflammatory drug (NSAID) limited to external use in ointment form. A trade name is Tanderil.

oxytetracycline – a broad-spectrum tetracycline antibiotic derived from the mould *Streptomyces rimosus*. The drug is effective against a range of germs including *Rickettsiae*. A trade name is Terramycin.

oxytocin – a natural hormone sometimes used as a drug to stimulate the muscle of the womb (uterus) and hasten childbirth.

Pacitron – a trade name for the antidepressant drug TRYPTOPHAN.

Painstop – a trade name for a compound of the painkiller drugs PARACETAMOL and CODEINE.

Paldesic – a trade name for PARACETAMOL.

Palfium – a trade name for DEXTROMORAMIDE.

Paludrine – a trade name for PROGUANIL.

Pamergan – a trade name for a compound of PETHIDINE and PROMETHAZINE.

Pameton – a trade name for a compound of PARACETAMOL and its antidote methionine.

Pamine – a trade name for HYOSCINE.

Panadeine – a trade name for a compound of PARACETAMOL and CODEINE.

Panadol – a trade name for PARACETAMOL.

Panamax – a trade name for PARACETAMOL.

Panasorb – a trade name for a readily absorbable form of PARACETAMOL.

Pancrease – a trade name for PANCREATIN.

pancreatin – a mixture of the digestive enzymes lipase, amylase and protease. The drug is used to treat people unable to digest fats and starches because of a deficiency of these enzymes. A trade name is Pancreatin Enseals.

Pancrex – a trade name for PANCREATIN.

Panoxyl – a trade name for BENZOYL PEROXIDE.

Pantheline – a trade name for PROPANTHELINE.

pantothenic acid – one of the B group of vitamins. Deficiency is rare.

papain – a mixture of enzymes found in papaya fruit. Papain includes the protein-splitting enzyme chymopapain and this makes it useful for breaking down organic debris and so cleaning up wounds and ulcers. Chymopapain is used to break down material extruded from the pulpy nuclei of intervertebral discs (chemonucleolysis).

papaveretum – a mixture of purified opium alkaloids. Papaveretum is mainly used for surgical premedication. A trade name is Omnopon.

papaverine – an opium derivative used as a smooth muscle relaxant and to treat heart irregularities following a heart attack. A trade name is Brovon.

paracetamol – a drug used to relieve minor pain (an analgesic drug) and to reduce fever. The real generic drug name is acetaminophen. The drug is widely used to relieve pain and reduce fever. It does not irritate the stomach, as Aspirin does, but overdose causes liver and kidney damage and may cause death from liver failure. 15 grams or more is potentially serious. The victim remains well for a day or two and liver failure develops between the third and fifth day. There are many trade names including Panadol, Anacin-3, Tempra and Tylenol.

Paradex – a trade name for a compound of DEXTROPROPOXYPHENE and PARACETAMOL.

paraldehyde – a rapidly acting drug used by injection to control severe excitement, delirium, mania or convulsions.

Paralgin – a trade name for PARACETAMOL.

Paraspen – a trade name for PARACETAMOL.

Parlodel – a trade name for BROMOCRIPTINE.

Parmid – a trade name for METOCLOPRAMIDE.

Parmol – a trade name for PARACETAMOL.

Parnate – a trade name for the antidepressant drug TRANYLCYPROMINE.

Parstelin – a trade name for a compound of TRANYLCYPROMINE and TRIFLUOPERAZINE.

Paxadon – a trade name for pyridoxine (vitamin B6).

Paxalgesic – a trade name for CO-PROXAMOL.

Paxane – a trade name for FLURAZEPAM.

Paxofen – a trade name for IBUPROFEN.

pemoline – a weak stimulant of the nervous system used to treat abnormal overactivity (the hyperkinetic syndrome) in children. It is taken by mouth. Possible side effects include headache, irritability, dizziness, sweating, palpitations, loss of appetite, weight loss and dry mouth. A trade name is Volital.

Penbritin – a trade name for AMPICILLIN.

Pendramine – a trade name for PENICILLAMINE.

penicillamine – a drug used to treat severe rheumatoid arthritis not responding to non-steroidal anti-inflammatory drugs (NSAIDs). A trade name is Cuprimine.

penicillin – one of an important group of antibiotic drugs. The original natural penicillin was derived from the mould *Penicillium* but the extensive range of penicillins in use nowadays is produced synthetically.

pentaerythitol tetranitrate – a drug used to relieve the symptoms of angina pectoris. A trade name is Mycardol.

Pentalgin – a trade name for a compound of PARACETAMOL, CODEINE and PENTOBARBITONE.

pentamidine – a drug effective against single-celled organisms (protozoa) and used in the treatment of *Pneumocystis carinii* pneumonia in AIDS, African sleeping sickness (trypanosomiasis) and a serious form of leishmaniasis (kala azar). It is administered by injection or from an inhaler. Possible side effects include low blood pressure, heart irregularity, low blood sugar (hypoglycaemia), low white blood cell count, pancreatitis and kidney damage. Trade names are Pentam 300, Nebupent.

pentazocine – a synthetic painkilling drug with actions similar to those of MORPHINE. A trade name is Fortral.

pentobarbitone – a now little-used BARBITURATE sedative and sleep-encouraging (hypnotic) drug of medium duration of action. Pentobarbitone is occasionally given as a premedication before surgery. A trade name is Nembutal.

Pentothal – a trade name for sodium THIOPENTONE.

Peptard – a trade name for HYOSCYAMINE.

Percutol – a trade name for GLYCERYL TRINITRATE in a formulation for absorption through the skin.

pergolide – a DOPAMINE receptor agonist drug used to help in the management of Parkinsonism. It is taken by mouth. Possible side effects include confusion, hallucinations, sleepiness, heart irregularity, nausea, breathing difficulties and double vision. A trade name is Celance.

Periactin – a trade name for the antihistamine and appetite-stimulating drug cyproheptadine.

Pernivit – a mixture of NICOTINIC ACID and acetomenaphthone, used to treat chilblains.

perphenazine – a phenothiazine derivative drug used in the treatment of schizophrenia and other psychotic conditions. It is also used to relieve severe vomiting and control persistent hiccups. A trade name is Fentazin.

Persantin – a trade name for the antiplatelet drug DIPYRIDAMOLE.

Pertofran – a trade name for the tricyclic antidepressant drug desipramine.

pethidine – a synthetic narcotic painkilling drug somewhat less powerful than MORPHINE. Pethidine is widely used during childbirth and as a premedication. Overuse may lead to addiction. Also known as meperidine or Demerol.

Pevaril – a trade name for the antifungal drug ECONAZOLE.

Phazyme – a trade name for the silicone preparation DIMETHICONE, used to treat indigestion from intestinal gas.

phencyclidine – a drug of abuse, commonly known as 'angel dust'. Also known as PCP.

phenelzine – an antidepressant drug of the monoamine oxidase inhibitor group. A trade name is Nardil.

Phenergan – a trade name for PROMETHAZINE.

phenformin – an oral hypoglycaemic agent formerly used in the control of maturity onset (Type II) diabetes but now withdrawn because of side effects.

phenindamine – an antihistamine drug used to treat allergic conditions. It is taken by mouth. Possible side effects include dry mouth, drowsiness and digestive upsets. A trade name is Thephorin.

phenindione – an anticoagulant drug that can be taken by mouth. Now little used because of allergic side effects. A trade name is Dindevan.

pheniramine – an antihistamine drug used to control allergic reactions. A trade name is Daneral.

phenmetrazine – an appetite-suppressant drug. A trade name is Preludin, Endurets.

phenobarbitone – a long-acting barbiturate drug now used mainly as an anticonvulsant. Phenobarbitone is no longer used as a sedative or sleep-encouraging (hypnotic) drug because its action is far too prolonged. A trade name is Luminal.

phenoxybenzamine – an alpha-adrenergic blocker drug with a powerful and persistent action, used to treat bladder neck obstruction and the effects of the adrenaline-producing tumour, the phaeochromocytoma. A trade name is Dibenyline.

phenoxymethylpenicillin – a synthetic PENICILLIN. A trade name is Crystapen V.

Phensedyl – a trade name for a compound of CODEINE, EPHEDRINE and PROMETHAZINE.

phentermine – a drug with an AMPHETAMINE-like action used for appetite control in obesity. A trade name is Duromine.

phentolamine – a drug used in the treatment of the adrenalin-producing tumour phaeochromocytoma.

phenylbutazone – a non-steroidal anti-inflammatory drug (NSAID) once widely used but now withdrawn from general prescription because of its tendency to cause heart failure from fluid retention and severe blood disorders. It is still used, under specialist supervision, in cases of ankylosing spondylitis (persistent inflammation and fixity of the spine). A trade name is Butazolidin.

phenylephrine – a decongestant drug commonly used to relieve the symptoms of hay fever (allergic rhinitis) and the common cold. A trade name is Hayphryn.

phenylpropanolamine – a decongestant drug used to treat the symptoms of hay fever (allergic rhinitis), sinusitis and the common cold. A trade name is Dimotapp LA.

phenytoin – an anti-epilepsy drug. A trade name is Dilantin.

pholcodine – an opioid drug used mainly for cough suppression.

Pholcomed – a trade name for a compound of PAPAVERINE and the cough suppressant PHOLCODINE.

pilocarpine – a drug used in the form of eye drops to treat glaucoma. Pilocarpine causes extreme constriction of the pupils. A trade name is Sno Pilo.

Pilopt – a trade name for eye drops containing PILOCARPINE.

pimozide – a long-acting phenothiazine antipsychotic drug that is also used in the treatment of the grunting and swearing Gilles de la Tourette's syndrome. A trade name is Orap.

pindolol – a beta-blocker drug used in the treatment of angina pectoris, high blood pressure and heart irregularity. Possible side effects include sleep disturbance, tiredness, digestive upset, cold hands and feet, asthma and undue slowing of the heart. A trade name is Visken.

piperazine – a deworming drug used to get rid of roundworms and threadworms. The drug paralyses the worms which are then passed with the faeces. A trade name is Antepar.

pirenzepine – a drug used to reduce secretion of acid by the stomach in the treatment of peptic ulcer. A trade name is Gastrozepin.

Piriton – a trade name for the antihistamine drug CHLORPHENIRAMINE.

piroxicam – a non-steroidal anti-inflammatory drug (NSAID) used mainly to control symptoms in the various forms of arthritis. A trade name is Feldene.

Pitressin – a trade name for VASOPRESSIN.

pivampicillin – a broad-spectrum penicillin-type antibiotic used to treat bronchitis, pneumonia, skin infections, urinary infections and gonorrhoea. It is taken by mouth. Possible side effects include allergic reactions, nausea and vomiting. A trade name is Pondocillin.

pivmecillinam – a penicillin-type antibiotic used to treat urinary infections and other infections with mecillinam-sensitive organisms. It is taken by mouth. Possible side effects include allergic reactions, nausea and vomiting. A trade name is Selexid.

pizotifen – an antihistamine drug used in the treatment of severe migraine. It is taken by mouth. Possible side effects include dizziness, drowsiness, increased appetite and weight gain, dry mouth, blurred vision and muscle pain. A trade name is Sanomigran.

Planequil – a trade name for the CHLOROQUINE-like antimalarial drug hydroxychloroquine.

Platamine – a trade name for CISPLATIN.

Platosin – a trade name for CISPLATIN.

podophyllin – a resin that may be applied locally in the treatment of various kinds of warts. Podophyllin is damaging to normal skin and must be applied with care.

Polybactrin – a trade name for a compound of the antibiotics BACITRACIN, NEOMYCIN and POLYMYXIN. For external use.

Polycrol – a trade name for a compound of the antacid drugs ALUMINIUM HYDROXIDE and MAGNESIUM HYDROXIDE and the antifoaming agent DIMETHICONE.

polymyxins – a group of five antibiotic drugs active against various unusual bacteria. They are used almost exclusively as external applications in ointments and eye and ear drops because of their toxicity if taken internally.

Polytar – a trade name for COAL TAR.

Ponderax – a trade name for the weight-control drug FENFLURAMINE.

Ponstan – a trade name for MEFENAMIC ACID.

potassium permanganate – a soluble compound that gives a skin-staining, deep purple solution with antiseptic and astringent properties.

Pragmatar – a trade name for a compound of coal tar, the skin-softening agent salicylic acid and sulphur.

Pramin – a trade name for METOCLOPRAMIDE.

Praminil – a trade name for IMIPRAMINE.

Praxilene – a trade name for the artery-widening (vasodilator) drug NAFTIDROFURYL.

praziquantel – a deworming (anthelmintic) drug used to dispose of tapeworms, schistosomes, liver flukes and lung flukes. It is taken by mouth. Possible side effects include nausea, abdominal discomfort, fever, sweating and drowsiness. A trade name is Biltricide.

prazosin – a drug that widens arteries (vasodilator) and is used in the treatment of high blood pressure, heart failure and Raynaud's phenomenon. A trade name is Hypovase.

Prednefrin Forte – a trade name for eye drops containing PREDNISOLONE and PHENYLEPHRINE.

Prednesol – a trade name for PREDNISOLONE.

prednisolone – a semisynthetic steroid drug derived from the natural steroid hormone cortisol and used in the treatment of a wide range of inflammatory disorders. A trade name is Predsol.

prednisone – a synthetic steroid drug used to reduce inflammation and relieve symptoms in rheumatoid arthritis, ulcerative colitis and many other conditions. A trade name is Decortisyl.

Predsol – a trade name for PREDNISOLONE.

Prefil – a trade name for the bulk-forming antidiarrhoeal agent sterculia.

Pregaday – a trade name for a compound of FOLIC ACID and IRON.

Premarin – a trade name for a preparation of oestrogens linked to other molecules (conjugated oestrogens). The name is said to derive from the source – pregnant mare's urine.

Prestim – a trade name for a compound of BENDROFLUAZIDE and TIMOLOL.

Priadel – a trade name for LITHIUM.

primaquine – a drug used in the treatment of *Plasmodium vivax* and *Plasmodium ovale* malaria.

primidone – an anticonvulsant drug used in the treatment of epilepsy. A trade name is Mysoline.

Primodian – a trade name for a preparation of the male sex hormone TESTOSTERONE.

Primogyn – a trade name for a preparation of the female sex hormone OESTRADIOL.

Primolut N – a trade name for NORETHISTERONE.

Primoteston – a trade name for TESTOSTERONE.

Primperan – a trade name for METOCLOPRAMIDE.

Pripsen – a trade name for a compound of the deworming drug PIPERAZINE and the laxative senna.

Pro-Actidil – a trade name for TRIPROLIDINE.

Pro-Banthine – a trade name for the antispasmodic drug PROPANTHELINE.

probenecid – a drug used in the treatment of gout. Probenecid acts by increasing the rate of excretion of uric acid in the urine and thus lowering its levels in the body. A trade name is Benemid.

probucol – a cholesterol-lowering drug. A trade name is Lurselle.

procainamide – a local anaesthetic-like drug used intravenously to control heart irregularities. It does this by its action to diminish the excitability of the specialized muscle cells in the heart muscle that transmit the stimulus to contract (conducting bundles). A trade name is Pronestyl.

procaine – a local anaesthetic drug now largely replaced by others that are more quickly effective or of more persistent action.

procarbazine – an anticancer drug used especially in the treatment of lymphomas. It is taken by mouth. Possible side effects include nausea and vomiting, loss of appetite and interference with bone marrow blood cell production. A trade name is Natulan.

prochlorperazine – a phenothiazine derivative antipsychotic drug used to treat schizophrenia and mania and to relieve nausea and vomiting. A trade name is Stemetil.

procyclidine – an anti-nerve-stimulating drug used to treat Parkinson's disease. A trade name is Arpicolin.

Prodexin – a trade name for the antacid drug MAGNESIUM CARBONATE.

Proflex – a trade name for IBUPROFEN.

Progesic – a trade name for FENOPROFEN.

progesterone – a steroid hormone produced mainly by the corpus luteum in the ovary that prepares the lining of the womb (uterus) for pregnancy.

Progout – a trade name for ALLOPURINOL.

proguanil – an antimalarial drug mainly used for prevention (as a prophylactic). A trade name is Paludrine.

promazine – a phenothiazine derivative antipsychotic drug used as a sedative. A trade name is Sparine.

promethazine – an antihistamine drug used to relieve itching, to control motion sickness and as a sedative. A trade name is Phenergan.

Prominal – a trade name for the barbiturate drug METHYLPHENOBARBITONE.

Prondol – a trade name for IPRINDOL.

Pronestyl – a trade name for PROCAINAMIDE.

propantheline – an antispasmodic drug used to relieve bowel spasm and to treat the irritable bowel syndrome and urinary incontinence caused by an irritable bladder. A trade name is Pro-Banthine.

propoxyphene – a painkilling drug. A trade name is Darvon.

propranolol – a beta-blocker drug used to treat high blood pressure (hypertension), angina pectoris and heart irregularities. Possible side effects include sleep disturbance, tiredness, digestive upset, cold hands and feet, asthma and undue slowing of the heart. A trade name is Inderal.

propylthiouracil – a drug used to treat overactivity of the thyroid gland (hyperthyroidism).

prostaglandin – one of a range of synthetic forms of the natural prostaglandin hormones such as DINOPROST.

Prostigmin – a trade name for NEOSTIGMINE.

protamine zinc insulin – a slow-release form of insulin with an action lasting for 12–24 hours. A trade name is Humulin Zn.

Protaphane – a trade name for a form of INSULIN.

Prothezine – a trade name for PROMETHAZINE.

Prothiaden – a trade name for DOTHIEPIN.

prothionamide – a drug used in the treatment of tuberculosis resistant to commoner drugs.

Protran – a trade name for CHLORPROMAZINE.

protriptyline – an antidepressant drug used especially to treat narcolepsy (sudden periods of very deep sleep) or depression associated with pathological lethargy (an abnormal degree of tiredness). A trade name is Concordin.

Pro-Vent – a trade name for THEOPHYLLINE.

Provera – a trade name for the progesterone-like drug METHYLPROGESTERONE.

Pro-Viron – a trade name for the male sex hormone drug MESTEROLONE.

Psoradrate – a trade name for a compound of the antipsoriasis drug DITHRANOL and urea.

psoralen – a plant derivative (coumarin) which, when applied to the skin or taken internally, increases the tendency of the skin to pigment under the action of ultraviolet light. This effect is exploited in the treatment of psoriasis and other skin conditions.

Psorin – a trade name for a compound of the antipsoriasis drug DITHRANOL, COAL TAR and the skin-softening agent SALICYLIC ACID.

Pulmadil – a trade name for the bronchodilator drug RIMITEROL.

Puri-Nethol – a trade name for MERCAPTOPURINE.

pyrantel – a deworming (anthelmintic) drug used to treat intestinal worm infestations, especially roundworms and threadworms. It is taken by mouth. Side effects occur only with large doses and include headache, dizziness, skin rash and fever. A trade name is Antiminth, Combantrin.

pyrazinamide – an antituberculous drug that diffuses well into the cerebrospinal fluid and is used to treat tuberculous meningitis. It is taken by mouth. Possible side effects include liver damage. A trade name is Rifater.

pyrazolones – a group of non-steroidal anti-inflammatory drugs (NSAIDs) that includes PHENYLBUTAZONE and AZAPROPAZONE.

pyridostigmine – a nerve-stimulating acetylcholine-like drug (see Chapter 3 – anticholinergic drugs). It acts by interfering with the enzyme that breaks down acetylcholine. It is used in the treatment of the muscle-weakening disease myasthenia gravis. It is taken by mouth or given by injection. Possible side effects include nausea, vomiting, abdominal pain, diarrhoea, sweating and increased salivation. A trade name is Mestinon.

pyridoxine – one of the B_6 group of vitamins. Deficiency is rare.

pyrimethamine – a drug used in the treatment of malaria and the protozoal disease toxoplasmosis. It is taken by mouth. Possible side effects include loss of appetite and vomiting. A trade name is Daraprim.

pyrithioxine – a vitamin B_6 derivative said to be useful in the management of senile dementia and behavioural disorders in children.

Pyrogastrone – a trade name for a compound of the antacid drugs ALUMINIUM HYDROXIDE, SODIUM BICARBONATE and MAGNESIUM TRISILICATE, the antifoaming agent alginic acid and the ulcer-protective drug CARBENOXOLONE.

qinghaosu – a drug derived from a Chinese medicinal herb qing hao (*Artemisia annua*) that has been found to be remarkably effective against malaria. Many trials have suggested that the drug cures malaria more rapidly than existing antimalarial drugs. Qinghaosu compounds appear to be almost non-toxic. The drug is still being evaluated in the West.

quinacrine – a yellow acridine dye useful in studying chromosomal structure because of its property of fluorescing when bound to certain regions of chromosomes. Also known as mepacrine. Quinacrine was once widely used to prevent malaria and to remove tapeworms.

Quinate – a trade name for QUININE.

Quinbisul – a trade name for QUININE.

Quinidex SA – a trade name for QUINIDINE.

quinidine – a drug derived from QUININE and used to control irregularity or excessive rapidity of the heart beat by depressing the excitability of the muscle. Trade names are Cardioquin, Quinidex SA and Quinidoxin.

Quinidoxin – a trade name for QUINIDINE.

quinine – the first drug found to be effective in the prevention and treatment of malaria. Quinine was originally derived from the bark of the cinchona tree. It is still used to treat CHLOROQUINE-resistant malaria but is no longer used as a preventive (prophylactic). Trade names are Quinoctal and Quinsul.

Quinoctal – a trade name for QUININE.

Quinsul – a trade name for QUININE.

Rafen – a trade name for IBUPROFEN.

ranitidine – a histamine receptor antagonist drug used to reduce acid secretion in cases of peptic ulceration. A trade name is Zantac.

Rapidard – a trade name for a preparation of INSULIN.

rauwolfia – dried extracts from the plant *Rauwolfia serpentina* that contains the alkaloid RESERPINE, a sedative and tranquillizing drug that also lowers blood pressure.

Redoxon – vitamin C.

Refrane – a trade name for LOBELINE.

Renitec – a trade name for ENALAPRIL.

reserpine – a RAUWOLFIA alkaloid that decreases the concentration of the nerve stimulator (neurotransmitter) 5-hydroxytryptamine in the nervous system and has a sedative and tranquillizing effect and lowers blood pressure. The drug has now been largely replaced by later and better antipsychotic drugs.

Respolin – a trade name for SALBUTAMOL.

Resprim – a trade name for CO-TRIMOXAZOLE.

Retin A – a trade name for TRETINOIN.

retinol – the common form of vitamin A found in animal and fish livers and other foods of animal origin. It is easily converted in the body into the active form, retinal.

Retrovir – a trade name for an antiviral drug with some useful effect against the retrovirus HIV that causes AIDS. Also known as AZT (azidothymidine) and ZIDOVUDINE.

Rheumacin – a trade name for INDOMETHACIN.

ribavirin – see TRIBAVIRIN.

riboflavin – vitamin B_2.

Rifadin – a trade name for RIFAMPICIN.

rifampicin – an antibiotic drug used mainly to treat tuberculosis and leprosy, but also Legionnaire's disease, inflammation of the prostate gland (prostatitis), inflammation of the lining of the heart (endocarditis) and inflammation of the bone marrow (osteomyelitis). Rifampicin interferes with the action of oral contraceptives. It is taken by mouth. Possible side effects include skin rashes, influenza-like symptoms, and digestive upset. Trade names include Tifadin, Rimycin, Rimactane.

rimiterol – an air-tube widening (bronchodilator) drug used in the treatment of asthma and bronchitis. It is taken by inhalation from an inhaler. Possible side effects include headaches and flushing. A trade name is Pulmadil.

Rimycin – a trade name for RIFAMPICIN.

ritodrine – a drug that relaxes the muscles of the womb and is used to prevent the onset of premature labour. A trade name is Yutopar.

Rivotril – a trade name for CLONAZEPAM.

royal jelly – a foodstuff secreted by worker bees for the nutrition of larvae and queen bees. The substance has been recommended for various disorders but there is no reason to suppose that royal jelly has any medicinal value.

RU486 – see MIFEPRISTONE.

Rynacrom – a trade name for CROMOGLYCATE.

Rythmodan – a trade name for DISOPYRAMIDE.

Sabin vaccine – an effective oral vaccine used to immunize against poliomyelitis. This vaccine contains live viruses that have been made safe. These spread by faecal contamination of food in the manner of the original disease, thus effectively extending the protection.

Salazopyrin – a trade name for the drug SULPHASALAZINE used to treat rheumatoid arthritis, ulcerative colitis and Crohn's disease.

Salbulin – a trade name for SALBUTAMOL.

salbutamol – an air-tube widening (bronchodilator) drug used to treat asthma, chronic bronchitis and emphysema. It is also sometimes used to relax the muscle of the womb and prevent premature labour. It is taken by mouth or by inhalation from an inhaler. Possible side effects include headache, anxiety, tremor and flushing. A trade name is Volmax.

salicylates – a group of anti-inflammatory, mildly painkilling and fever-reducing (antipyretic) drugs that includes Aspirin, SODIUM SALICYLATE and BENORYLATE.

salicylic acid – a drug that softens and loosens the horny outer layer of the skin (the epidermis) and is used in the treatment of various skin disorders such as psoriasis, ichthyosis, warts and callosities.

Salk vaccine – a killed virus antipoliomyelitis vaccine.

salmeterol – a new anti-asthma drug, taken by inhalation, that produces widening of the air tubes for at least 12 hours. Salmeterol acts by causing long-term stimulation of the receptors (beta-2 adrenoceptors) that relax the bronchial tube muscles.

salsalate – a non-steroidal anti-inflammatory drug (NSAID).

Saluric – a trade name for the drug CHLOROTHIAZIDE.

Sandimmun – a trade name for CYCLOSPORIN.

Sandocal – a trade name for a calcium preparation.

Savlon – a trade name for a CETRIMIDE preparation.

Scop – a trade name for HYOSCINE.

scopolamine – an ATROPINE-like drug used in premedication as a sedative and to dry up respiratory and salivary secretions.

Seconal – a trade name for a barbiturate drug now seldom prescribed.

Sectral – a trade name for ACEBUTOLOL.

Securon – a trade name for the drug VERAPAMIL.

selegiline – a selective mono-amine-oxidase inhibitor drug used in the treatment of Parkinsonism. Selegiline is thought to retard the breakdown of DOPAMINE. It is taken by mouth. Possible side effects include fainting on standing up, involuntary movements, nausea or confusion. A trade name is Eldepryl.

selenium – a trace element recently found to be an essential component of the enzyme deiodinase which catalyzes the production of tri-iodothyronine (T3) from thyroxine (T4) in the thyroid gland. Selenium deficiency prevents the formation of T3. Selenium sulphide is a selenium compound used to treat dandruff. It is administered in a shampoo. Trade names are Lenium, Selsun.

Selsun – a trade name for a SELENIUM-containing shampoo used to treat dandruff.

Semitard MC – a trade name for a form of INSULIN having medium duration of action.

Septrin – a trade name for the antibacterial drug CO-TRIMOXAZOLE.

Serc – a trade name for the drug BETAHISTINE.

Serenace – a trade name for the tranquillizing drug HALOPERIDOL.

Serepax – a trade name for OXAZEPAM.

Serophene – a trade name for the drug CLOMIPHENE.

Sigmacort – a trade name for HYDROCORTISONE.

Simeco – a trade name for a compound of the antacids aluminium hydroxide and magnesium hydroxide and the antifoaming agent SIMETHICONE.

simethicone – a silicone-based material with antifoaming properties used in the treatment of flatulence and often incorporated into antacid remedies. Simethicone is also used as a water-repellent skin-protecting agent in the management of nappy rash and other skin disorders.

Sinequan – a trade name for the tranquillizing drug DOXEPIN.

Sintisone – a trade name for PREDNISOLONE.

Sinutab Antihistamine – a trade name for a compound of PARACETAMOL, PSEUDOEPHEDRINE and CHLORPHENIRAMINE.

Sinuzets – a trade name for capsules containing PARACETAMOL, PSEUDOEPHEDRINE and PHENYLEPHRINE.

Skitz – a trade name for BENZOYL PEROXIDE.

Slow-Bid – a trade name for THEOPHYLLINE.

Slow-Fe – a trade name for an IRON preparation.

Slo-K – a trade name for a POTASSIUM preparation.

sodium aurothiomalate – a gold preparation given by injection for the treatment of rheumatoid arthritis.

sodium bicarbonate – baking soda. An antacid drug used to relieve indigestion, heartburn and the pain of peptic ulcer. Sodium bicarbonate is not a preferred antacid as it leads to the production of carbon dioxide and 'rebound' acid production.

sodium pentothal – a rapid-acting barbiturate drug used for the induction of general anaesthesia.

sodium salicylate – a painkilling drug used to treat rheumatic fever. It has no advantages over Aspirin (acetyl salicylic acid) and the same adverse effects.

sodium valproate – an anticonvulsant drug used to treat epilepsy.

Sofradex – a trade name for eye or ear drops or ointment containing DEXAMETHASONE, FRAMYCETIN and GRAMICIDIN.

Soframycin – a trade name for the antibiotic drug FRAMYCETIN.

Solcode – a trade name for a compound of Aspirin and CODEINE.

Solone – a trade name for PREDNISOLONE.

Solprin – a trade name for Aspirin.

Solu-Cortef – a trade name for HYDROCORTISONE.

Solu-Medrol – a trade name for METHYLPREDNISOLONE.

somatrem – a preparation of human growth hormone used to treat short stature caused by growth hormone deficiency.

Sominex – a trade name for the antihistamine drug PROMETHAZINE used as a sedative.

Somophyllin – a trade name for AMINOPHYLLINE.

Sone – a trade name for PREDNISONE.

Soneryl – a trade name for the barbiturate drug BUTOBARBITONE.

sorbitol – a sweetening agent derived from glucose.

sotalol – a long-acting beta-blocker drug used to treat irregularity of the heart action. Possible side effects include sleep disturbance, tiredness, digestive upset, cold hands and feet, asthma and undue slowing of the heart. A trade name is Beta-Cardone.

Span K – a trade name for a potassium preparation.

Spanish fly – dried extract of the blister beetle, *Lytta vesicatoria*. Cantharides. This is a highly irritant and poisonous substance with an unjustified reputation as an aphrodisiac.

Sparine – a trade name for PROMAZINE.

Spiretic – a trade name for SPIRONOLACTONE.

spironolactone – a urine-promoting (diuretic) drug that does not lead to loss of potassium from the body. It is an antagonist of the hormone aldosterone. A trade name is Aldactone.

Stafoxil – a trade name for the antibiotic FLUCLOXACILLIN.

stanozolol – an anabolic steroid drug used to treat the effects of deep vein thrombosis and the tissue-hardening disease systemic sclerosis. A trade name is Stromba.

Staphlipen – a trade name for the antibiotic FLUCLOXACILLIN.

Staphylex – a trade name for FLUCLOXACILLIN.

Stelazine – a trade name for TRIFLUOPERAZINE.

Stemetil – a trade name for PROCHLORPERAZINE.

stilboestrol – a synthetic oestrogen drug similar in action to the natural hormone oestradiol. Stilboestrol is used to treat cancer of the prostate gland, some types of breast cancer and post-menopausal wasting (atrophy) of the vaginal wall. A trade name is Tampovagan.

Streptase – a trade name for STREPTOKINASE.

streptokinase – protein-splitting enzyme used as a drug to dissolve blood clots in a coronary artery so as to minimize the degree of heart muscle death (myocardial infarction) during a heart attack. It is also used to treat blood clots blocking the lung arteries (pulmonary embolism).

streptomycin – an aminoglycoside antibiotic drug used to treat some rare infections such as brucellosis, glanders, plague, tuberculosis and tularaemia. It is administered by injection but is avoided for commoner infections because of its side effects, which include deafness and tinnitus.

strychnine – a bitter-tasting, highly poisonous substance occurring in the seeds of *Strychnos* species of tropical trees and shrubs. Poisoning causes restlessness, stiffness of the face and neck, exaggerated sensations, extreme arching of the back (opisthotonus) and death from paralysis of breathing unless artificial ventilation is used.

sucralfate – an aluminium-containing drug that forms a protective coating over the lining of the stomach or the immediately following section of bowel (the duodenum). Sucralfate is used in the treatment of peptic ulcer. It is taken by mouth. A fairly common side effect is constipation. A trade name is Antepsin.

Sudafed – a trade name for PSEUDOEPHEDRINE.

sulfadoxine – a sulphonamide drug used as an adjunct to CHLOROQUINE in the treatment of *Falciparum* malaria. A trade name is Fansidar.

sulindac – a non-steroidal anti-inflammatory drug (NSAID). A trade name is Clinoril.

sulphacetamide – a sulphonamide drug limited to external use, as in eye drops for the treatment of conjunctivitis. A trade name is Albucid.

sulphadiazine – a readily absorbed and quickly eliminated sulphonamide drug used in mixtures with other similar drugs in the treatment of various infections, especially urinary infections.

sulphasalazine – a compound of a sulphonamide drug and 5-aminosalicylic acid used to treat rheumatoid arthritis, ulcerative colitis and Crohn's disease. A trade name is Salazopyrin.

sulphamethoxazole – a sulphonamide drug still widely used in combination with TRIMETHOPRIM to provide a combination highly effective against infections of the urinary system and respiratory system. It is taken by mouth. Possible side effects include drug rashes and a rare but serious skin and eye disorder known as the Stevens-Johnson syndrome. A trade name, with trimethoprim is Septrin.

sulphinpyrazone – a drug that promotes the loss of uric acid in the urine (a uricosuric drug) used to reduce the frequency of attacks of gout. A trade name is Anturan.

sulpiride – an antipsychotic drug used to treat acute and long-term schizophrenic illness. It is taken by mouth. Possible side effects include muscle spasm, uncontrollable movements, restlessness and dry mouth. Trade names are Dolmatil, Sulpitil.

Sulpitil – a trade name for the antipsychotic drug SULPIRIDE.

sumatriptan – a serotonin antagonist drug that has been found effective in the symptomatic treatment of acute migraine. It is taken by mouth or given by injection. Possible side effects include dizziness, drowsiness, fatigue, chest pain and a rise in blood pressure. A trade name is Imigran.

Supradyn – a trade name for a multivitamin and mineral preparation.

suramin – a drug used in the treatment of African sleeping sickness (trypanosomiasis).

Surem – a trade name for the benzodiazepine drug NITRAZEPAM.

surfactant – a substance that reduces surface tension and promotes wetting of surfaces. The lungs contain a surfactant to prevent collapse of the tiny air sacs in the lungs (alveoli).

Surmontil – a trade name for the tricyclic antidepressant drug TRIMIPRAMINE.

Suscard – a trade name for the artery-widening drug GLYCERYL TRINITRATE (nitroglycerine).

Sustac – a trade name for the artery-widening drug GLYCERYL TRINITRATE (nitroglycerine).

Sustamycin – a trade name for the antibiotic TETRACYCLINE.

Sustanon – a trade name for the male sex hormone drug TESTOSTERONE.

Synanalar – a trade name for the steroid drug FLUOCINOLONE, used for local applications.

Synflex – a trade name for NAPROXEN.

Syntaris – a trade name for the steroid drug FLUNISOLIDE.

Syntocinon – a trade name for the womb (uterus) muscle stimulating drug OXYTOCIN.

syntopressin – a synthetic form, lypression, of the natural watercontrolling hormone vasopressin. This drug is used in the treatment of a disease in which there is excessive loss of water from the kidneys (diabetes insipidus). See VASOPRESSIN.

Syraprim – a trade name for the antibacterial drug TRIMETHOPRIM.

Sytron – a trade name for the iron preparation, sodium iron edetate, used in the treatment of anaemia.

tacrin – a shortened name for the drug TETRAHYDROAMINOACRIDINE.

Tagamet – a trade name for CIMETIDINE.

talampicillin – a penicillin type antibiotic of the AMPICILLIN ester class, effective against a wide range of bacteria. Talampicillin achieves higher blood concentrations than ampicillin. It is taken by mouth. A possible side effect is a severe penicillin hypersensitivity reactions.

Tamofen – a trade name for TAMOXIFEN.

tamoxifen – a drug that blocks oestrogen receptors and is useful in the treatment of certain cancers, especially breast cancer. It also stimulates egg production from the ovaries and can be used to treat infertility. Trade names are Nolvadex, Tamofen.

taxol – an anticancer drug formerly obtainable only from the bark of the Pacific yew tree but now synthesized. It has also been produced by biotechnological plant tissue culture methods. Taxol interacts with tubulin, a contractile protein involved in cell division and has been found to exercise control on the growth of ovarian, breast and lung cancers. Its use remains experimental.

Tegretol – a trade name for CARBAMAZEPINE.

Teldane – a trade name for TERFENADINE.

Temaze – a trade name for TEMAZEPAM.

temazepam – a benzodiazepine sedative drug of intermediate duration of action used to treat insomnia. It is taken by mouth. Possible side effects include confusion, vertigo, digestive upsets and skin rashes. Trade names are Normison, Temaze.

Temgesic – a trade name for BUPRENORPHINE.

Tempra – a trade name for PARACETAMOL.

Tenopt – a trade name for eye drops containing TIMOLOL.

Tenormin – a trade name for ATENOLOL.

Tensium – a trade name for DIAZEPAM.

Tenuate dospan – a trade name for the appetite-reducing drug DIETHYLPROPION.

terbutaline – an air-tube widening (bronchodilator) drug used in the treatment of asthma, bronchitis and emphysema. It is also used to relax the muscle of the womb and prevent premature labour. A trade name is Bricanyl.

terfenadine – an antihistamine drug used to treat hay fever (allergic rhinitis) and nettle rash (urticaria). It is taken by mouth. Possible side effects include headache, digestive upset, skin rashes, sweating and heart irregularity. A trade name is Triludan.

terlipressin – a drug that releases VASOPRESSIN over a period of hours. This is used to help to control bleeding from varicose veins of the gullet (oesophageal varices) by constricting the small arteries in the intestinal tract.

Terramycin – the tetracycline antibiotic OXYTETRACYCLINE.

Testomet – a trade name for METHYLTESTOSTERONE.

testosterone – the principal male sex hormone (androgen) produced in the testicles and, to a lesser extent in the ovary. Testosterone is anabolic and stimulates bone and muscle growth and the development of the sexual characteristics. It is also used as a drug to treat delayed puberty and some cases of infertility.

tetracaine hydrochloride – a local anaesthetic drug.

tetracosactrin – a substance similar to the pituitary gland adrenal-stimulating hormone ACTH. It is used as a test of adrenal function. An injection of the drug is given and the resulting rise in serum cortisol is monitored.

tetracycline – one of a group of antibiotic drugs used to treat a wide range of infections including rickettsial diseases, cholera, brucellosis and most of the sexually transmitted diseases. Trade names include Achromycin, Sumycin, Tetracyn.

tetrahydroaminoacridine – a drug that has been used experimentally to try to improve the situation of people with Alzheimer's disease.

Tetrex – a trade name for TETRACYCLINE.

thalidomide – a drug (Distaval) that was widely advertised as a safe sedative. In 1961 it was found that, when given to pregnant women, it caused severe bodily malformation of the fetus with stunting of the limbs, which were often replaced by short flippers (phocomelia). Thalidomide has since been found useful in the treatment of certain forms of leprosy and Behçet's syndrome.

Theo-Dur – a trade name for THEOPHYLLINE.

theophylline – an air-tube widening (bronchodilator) drug used to treat asthma and to assist in the treatment of heart failure by increasing the heart rate and reducing water-logging (oedema) by promoting excretion of urine. Trade names are Franol, Theograd.

Thephorin – a trade name for PHENINDAMINE.

Theraderm – a trade name for the anti-acne drug BENZOYL PEROXIDE.

thiabendazole – a deworming drug used to get rid of worms such as *Toxocara canis*, *Strongyloides stercoralis* and *Trichinella spiralis*. A trade name is Mintezol.

thiacetazone – a drug used in conjunction with ISONIAZID in the treatment of tuberculosis.

thiamine – vitamin B$_1$.

thiethylperazine – a phenothiazine drug used to control severe nausea and vomiting. It is taken by mouth or given by injection. Possible side effects include drowsiness, involuntary movements, low blood pressure and nervous system disturbances. A trade name is Torecan.

thioguanine – a drug used in the treatment of acute myeloblastic leukaemia.

thiomersal – a mercurial antiseptic often used to sterilize eye drops and other solutions. Also known as thimerosal.

thiopentone – a barbiturate drug widely used as a pleasant and rapid induction agent for general anaesthesia. The drug is given by slow intravenous injection. A trade name is Pentothal.

Thioprine – a trade name for AZATHIOPRINE.

thioridazine – an antipsychotic drug used to treat schizophrenia and mania. A trade name is Melleril.

thiouracil – a drug that blocks the synthesis of thyroid hormone and can be used to treat thyroid overactivity.

thymoxamine – a drug that widens blood vessels (vasodilator) and may be useful in the management of spasm of the finger arteries (Raynaud's disease). A trade name is Opilon.

thyroxine – the principal thyroid hormone. Thyroxine has four iodine atoms in the molecule and is often known as T4.

tiaprofenic acid – a non-steroidal anti-inflammatory drug (NSAID).

ticarcillin – a PENICILLIN antibiotic useful for its action against the organism *Pseudomonas aeruginosa*.

Ticillin – a trade name for TICARCILLIN.

Tiempe – a trade name for TRIMETHOPRIM.

Tildiem – a trade name for DILTIAZEM.

timolol – a beta-blocker drug used to treat high blood pressure and angina pectoris and, in the form of eye drops, to treat glaucoma. Possible side effects (oral preparation) include sleep disturbance, tiredness, digestive upset, cold hands and feet, asthma and undue slowing of the heart. Trade names are Betim, Timoptol.

Timoptol – a trade name for eye drops containing the beta-blocker drug TIMOLOL, used to control glaucoma.

Tinacidin – a trade name for TOLNAFTATE.

Tinaderm-M – a trade name for a compound of the antifungal drugs NYSTATIN and TOLNAFTATE, used to treat skin fungal infections.

tinidazole – an antibacterial and antiprotozoal drug similar to METRONIDAZOLE but with a longer duration of action. Protozoa are microscopic single-celled animals that cause many human diseases. They include the organisms that cause amoebic dysentery, trichomonas infections, giardiasis, leishmaniasis, sleeping sickness and malaria.

Tinset – a trade name for the antihistamine drug OXATOMIDE.

Tobralex – a trade name for eye drops containing TOBRAMYCIN.

tobramycin – an antibiotic drug similar in use to GENTAMICIN, but useful in the treatment of gentamicin-resistant infections. A trade name is Nebcin.

tocainide – a drug used to treat a life-threatening tendency to cardiac arrest (ventricular fibrillation). It is taken by mouth. Possible side effects include nausea, vomiting, dizziness, tremor and reduced white blood cell production. A trade name is Tonocard.

tocopherol – one of the constituents of vitamin E.

Tofranil – a trade name for IMIPRAMINE.

Tolanase – a trade name for the oral antidiabetic drug TOLAZAMIDE.

tolazamide – a sulphonylurea drug used to treat maturity-onset, non-insulin-dependent diabetes.

tolazoline – a drug that causes marked dilatation of blood vessels and is used to treat conditions, such as Raynaud's disease in which blood vessels go into spasm.

tolbutamide – a drug used in the treatment of maturity-onset, non-insulin-dependent diabetes. A trade name is Rastinon.

Tolectin – a trade name for TOLMETIN.

tolmetin – a non-steroidal anti-inflammatory drug (NSAID) used especially for the relief of pain and stiffness in osteoarthritis, rheumatoid arthritis and ankylosing spondylitis. A trade name is Tolectin.

tolnaftate – an antifungal drug used to treat foot and body fungal infections (tinea). A trade name is Tinacidin.

Tonocard – a trade name for the antiarrhythmic heart drug TOCAINIDE.

Topal – a trade name for a compound of ALUMINIUM HYDROXIDE, ALGINIC ACID and MAGNESIUM CARBONATE, used to treat indigestion (dyspepsia).

Topilar – a trade name for the steroid drug FLUCLOROLONE, used for local (topical) applications.

Torecan – a trade name for the antivomiting (antiemetic) drug THIETHYLPERAZINE.

Trancopal – a trade name for CHLORMEZANONE.

Trandate – the beta-blocker drug LABETALOL.

trandolapril – an angiotensin converting enzyme (ACE) inhibitor drug used to treat high blood pressure. It is taken by mouth. Possible side effects include faintness, headache, dizziness, palpitations and skin rashes. A trade name is Gopten.

tranexamic acid – a drug used to control the breakdown of blood clots in the circulation and thus limit bleeding (an antifibrinolytic drug). It is taken by mouth. Possible side effects include nausea and vomiting. A trade name is Cyklokapron.

Tranxene – a trade name for CLORAZEPATE.

tranylcypromine – a monoamine-oxidase inhibitor antidepressant drug.

Trasicor – the beta-blocker drug OXPRENOLOL.

tretinoin – a drug used to treat acne and scaly skin conditions such as ichthyosis. A trade name is Retin-A.

triamcinolone – a steroid drug used to treat inflammatory disorders, asthma, shortage of blood platelets required for blood clotting (thrombocytopenia) and some forms of leukaemia. A trade name is Adcortyl.

triamterene – a potassium-sparing urine-promoting (diuretic) drug used to relieve the body of excess water and to treat mildly raised blood pressure. A trade name is Dytide.

triazolam – a benzodiazepine sedative drug used to relieve insomnia. A trade name is Halcion.

Trib – a trade name for CO-TRIMOXAZOLE.

tribavirin – an antiviral drug effective against a range of both DNA and RNA (ribonucleic acid) viruses including the herpes group and those causing hepatitis, several strains of influenza and Lassa fever. It is administered by a small-particle aerosol inhaler and sometimes by intravenous injection. Possible side effects include breathing difficulty, bacterial pneumonia and lung collapse (pneumothorax). Unfortunately, it antagonizes the action of zidovudine (AZT) against HIV. Trade names are Virax, Virazole.

trichlormethiazide – a urine-promoting (diuretic) drug also used to treat high blood pressure. A trade name is Diurese.

Trichozole – a trade name for METRONIDAZOLE.

Tridesilon – the steroid drug desonide, used for local applications.

Tridil – a trade name for GLYCERYL TRINITRATE.

trifluoperazine – a phenothiazine antipsychotic and antivomiting (antiemetic) drug used mainly to treat schizophrenia. It is taken by mouth. Possible side effects include restlessness, random uncontrollable movements, dry mouth, urinary retention and weight gain. A trade name is Stelazine.

trifluperidol – an antipsychotic drug with similar action to the phenothiazine derivative drugs. A trade name is Triperidol.

Trilafon – a trade name for PERPHENAZINE.

Triludan – the antihistamine drug TERFENADINE.

trimeprazine – an antihistamine drug used to relieve itching in allergic conditions and as a sedative for children. A trade name is Vallergan.

trimethoprim – an antibacterial drug commonly used to treat urinary infections. Combined with SULPHAMETHOXAZOLE it is sold as co-trimoxazole (Septrin). A trade name is Bactrim.

trimipramine – a tricyclic antidepressant drug with a strong sedative effect. It is taken by mouth. Possible side effects include constipation, blurred vision, dryness of the mouth and difficulty in urinating. A trade name is Surmontil.

Trimogal – a trade name for TRIMETHOPRIM.

Triominic – a mixture of the nasal decongestant drug PHENYLPROPANOLAMINE and the antihistamine drug PHENIRAMINE.

Triperidol – the antipsychotic drug TRIFLUPERIDOL.

triple vaccine – a combined vaccine against diphtheria, whooping cough (pertussis) and tetanus.

Triplopen – a combination of the three PENICILLIN antibiotics benethamine penicillin, procaine penicillin and BENZYLPENICILLIN.

Triprim – a trade name for TRIMETHOPRIM.

triprolidine – an antihistamine drug used to treat allergy and to relieve the symptoms of colds. Trade names are Actidil, Actifed.

Triptafen – a trade name for a compound of the tricyclic antidepressant drug AMITRIPTYLINE and the antipsychotic and antiemetic drug PERPHENAZINE.

tropicamide – a drug used in the form of eye drops to widen (dilate) the pupil so that the inside of the eye can more easily be examined or operated upon. A trade name is Mydriacyl.

Tropium – the benzodiazepine antianxiety drug CHLORDIAZEPOXIDE.

Tryptanol – a trade name for AMITRIPTYLINE.

Tryptizol – a trade name for AMITRIPTYLINE.

tryptophan – an antidepressant drug. L-tryptophan, sold in USA as a non-prescription food additive was withdrawn by the American Food and Drugs Administration (FDA) because of reports of a severe muscle disorder apparently caused by an unidentified contaminant. A trade name is Optimax.

Tussinol – a trade name for PHOLCODINE.

Tylex – a trade name for a compound of the painkilling drugs CODEINE and PARACETAMOL.

Tyrosets – a trade name for throat lozenges containing the local anaesthetic drug BENZOCAINE.

tyrothricin – an antibiotic obtained from the soil germ *Bacillus brevis* and used by local application to treat external infections. It is too poisonous for internal use.

Ukidan – a trade name for UROKINASE.

Ulcol – a trade name for SULPHASALAZINE.

Ultralente MC – a trade name for a long-acting form of INSULIN.

Ultratard – a trade name for a long-acting form of INSULIN.

Unicap T – a trade name for a multivitamin and mineral preparation.

Unihep – a trade name for the anticoagulant HEPARIN.

Unimycin – a trade name for the antibiotic drug OXYTETRACYCLINE.

Uniparin – a trade name for HEPARIN.

Unisomnia – a trade name for NITRAZEPAM.

Univer – a trade name for VERAPAMIL.

Urantoin – a trade name for the antibacterial drug NITROFURANTOIN.

Uremide – a trade name for FRUSEMIDE.

Urex – a trade name for FRUSEMIDE.

Uriben – a trade name for NALIDIXIC ACID.

Urisal – a trade name for sodium citrate, a drug used to make the urine less acid.

Urispas – a trade name for FLAVOXATE.

ursodeoxycholic acid – a drug used to treat cholesterol gallstones. It is taken by mouth. Side effects are infrequent but include diarrhoea and indigestion. Trade names are Destolit, Ursofalk.

Ursofalk – a trade name for URSODEOXYCHOLIC ACID.

Utovan – a trade name for NORETHISTERONE.

Vaginyl – a trade name for the drug METRONIDAZOLE.

Valcote – a trade name for SODIUM VALPROATE.

Valium – a trade name for DIAZEPAM.

Vallergan – a trade name for the antihistamine drug TRIMEPRAZINE.

Valoid – a trade name for CYCLIZINE.

valproic acid – an anti-epilepsy drug. A trade name is Depakote.

Vancocin – a trade name for VANCOMYCIN.

vancomycin – an antibiotic drug effective against many bacteria. It is poisonous and its use is limited to infections that fail to respond to the common antibiotics.

Varidase – a trade name for a compound of STREPTOKINASE and streptodornase used locally to remove blood clots and organic debris from wounds.

Vascardin – a trade name for ISOSORBIDE DINITRATE.

vasopressin – a natural pituitary gland hormone. Analogue substances, such as lypressin (pig vasopressin), terlipressin and desmopressin are used as drugs to treat deficiency of the natural hormone that causes the disorder diabetes insipidus. They are also used to treat dangerous bleeding from varicose veins in the gullet (oesophageal varices). These hormone analogues are administered by nasal spray or by injection. Possible side effects include abdominal cramps, headache and raised blood pressure. Trade names are Desmospray, Glypressin, Lypressin.

Veganin – a trade name for a compound of the painkilling drugs Aspirin, CODEINE and PARACETAMOL.

Velbe – a trade name for the anticancer drug VINBLASTINE.

Velosulin – a trade name for an INSULIN preparation.

venene – a mixture of snake venoms used to produce a general antidote (ANTIVENIN).

Ventide – a trade name for a compound of BECLOMETHASONE and SALBUTAMOL, used to control asthma.

Ventolin – a trade name for the bronchodilator drug SALBUTAMOL.

Veradil – a trade name for VERAPAMIL.

verapamil – a calcium channel blocker drug used to correct irregularities in the heart beat. Trade names are Calan, Cordilox, Securon, Univer.

Vermox – a trade name for the deworming drug MEBENDAZOLE.

Vibramycin – a trade name for DOXYCYCLINE.

vidarabine – a drug that inhibits DNA synthesis and is used to treat *Herpes simplex* (see Chapter 3 – herpes), shingles and a virus infection that results in great enlargement of invaded cells (cytomegalovirus infection). It is administered by intravenous infusion. Possible side effects are few but include weakness and skin rashes. A trade name is Vira-A.

vinblastine – an anticancer drug used mainly in the treatment of Hodgkin's disease and other lymphomas. Possible side effects include nausea and vomiting, loss of hair and interference with bone marrow blood cell production. A trade name is Velbe.

Vincent's powders – a trade name for Aspirin.

vincristine – a vinca alkaloid anticancer drug used to treat leukaemia. Possible side effects include nausea and vomiting, loss of hair and interference with bone marrow blood cell production. A trade name is Oncovin.

vindesine – a vinca alkaloid anticancer drug used to treat leukaemia. Possible side effects include nausea and vomiting, loss of hair and interference with bone marrow blood cell production. A trade name is Eldisine.

Viokase – a trade name for PANCREATIN.

viomycin – an antibiotic drug used in cases of tuberculosis that resist standard treatment.

Vira-A – a trade name for VIDARABINE.

Virormone – a trade name for the male sex hormone drug TESTOSTERONE.

Visclair – a trade name for METHYLCYSTEINE.

Visken – a trade name for PINDOLOL.

Visopt – a trade name for eye drops containing PHENYLEPHRINE and HYPROMELLOSE.

Voltaren, Voltarol – trade names for DICLOFENAC.

warfarin – an anticoagulant drug used to treat abnormal or undesired clotting of the blood. A trade name is Coumadin.

Welldorm – a trade name for the sleeping drug CHLORAL HYDRATE.

Wellferon – a trade name for an interferon preparation. Interferons are substances released by cells invaded by viruses that enable other cells to resist infection with viruses.

Winsprin – a trade name for Aspirin.

xamoterol – a beta-adrenergic agonist drug used in the treatment of long-term mild heart failure. It is taken by mouth. Possible side effects include headache, dizziness, muscle cramps, palpitations and skin rashes. A trade name is Corwin.

xipamide – a thiazide urine-promoting (diuretic) drug.

Xylocaine, Xylocard – trade names for the local anaesthetic drug LIGNOCAINE.

xylometazoline – a decongestant drug used to relieve a blocked nose.

yohimbin – an alkaloid adrenoreceptor antagonist derived from the yohimbe tree. It lowers blood pressure and controls arousal and anxiety and has been used to treat both physical and psychogenic impotence.

Yomesan – a trade name for the deworming drug NICLOSAMIDE.

Yutopar – a trade name for the womb-relaxing drug RITODRINE.

Zaditen – a trade name for the antiallergic drug KETOTIFEN.

Zadstat – a trade name for METRONIDAZOLE.

zalcitabine – a drug, similar to DIDANOSINE, that can block the action of the enzyme reverse transcriptase in the human immunodeficiency virus (HIV), the cause of AIDS. This action interferes with the replication of the virus in the human T cell. Zalcitabine cannot cure AIDS but is used to try to prolong life. It is taken by mouth. Possible side effects include reversible nerve damage, ulceration of the gullet, skin rashes, severe pancreatitis, nausea, vomiting and headache.

Zantac – a trade name for the stomach acid reducing drug RANITIDINE.

Zarontin – a trade name for ETHOSUXIMIDE.

zidovudine – an antiviral drug used to try to retard the progress of AIDS. Also known as azidothymidine or AZT. A trade name is Retrovir.

zimelidine – an antidepressant drug.

Zinamide – a trade name for PYRAZINAMIDE.

zinc oxide – a white powder with mild tissue-tightening (astringent) properties used as a dusting powder or incorporated into creams or ointments and used as a bland skin application. Mixed with oil of cloves, zinc oxide forms an effective and pain-relieving temporary dressing for a tooth cavity.

Zincaps – a trade name for a zinc preparation.

Zincfrin – a trade name for eye drops containing zinc sulphate and PHENYLEPHRINE.

Zinnat – a trade name for CEFUROXIME.

Zithromax – a trade name for AZITHROMYCIN.

Zofran – a trade name for ONDANSETRON.

Zonulysin – a trade name for the protein-splitting enzyme alpha-chymotrypsin. This is used in certain forms of cataract surgery when it is proposed to remove the whole of the cataractous lens from the eye. Zonulysin is made up in a solution that is run into the opened eye so that it can dissolving the fine suspensory fibres of the lens and allow easy removal of the lens with a freezing probe.

Zovirax – a trade name for the antiviral drug ACYCLOVIR.

Zyloprim – a trade name for ALLOPURINOL.

Zyloric – a trade name for ALLOPURINOL.

Zymafluor – a trade name for a fluoride preparation taken as a supplement when the local water supply provides inadequate quantities.

INDEX

COLLINS POCKET REFERENCE

phentermine. Duromine.